Manual of Systematic Corneal Surgery

Manual of Systematic Corneal Surgery

Arthur D McG Steele MB BS FRCS (Eng) FRACO FRCOphth

Consulting Ophthalmic Surgery, Moorfields Eye Hospital, London, UK

Colin M Kirkness BMedBiol MB ChB FRCS (Ed & Glas) FRCOphth

Tennent Professor of Ophthalmology, University of Glasgow, Glasgow, UK

Illustrations by **Terry Tarrant**

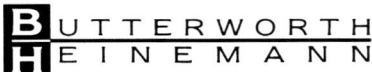

BUTTERWORTH
HEINEMANN

OXFORD AUCKLAND BOSTON JOHANNESBURG MELBOURNE NEW DELHI

Butterworth-Heinemann
Linacre House, Jordan Hill, Oxford OX2 8DP
225 Wildwood Avenue, Woburn, MA 01801-2041
A division of Reed Educational and Professional Publishing Ltd

℞ A member of the Reed Elsevier plc group

First published 1992 by Longman Group UK Limited

British Library Cataloguing in Publication Data
A catalogue record for this book is available from the British Library

Library of Congress Cataloguing in Publication Data
A catalogue record for this book is available from the Library of Congress

ISBN 0 7506 3720 X

Data manipulation by David Gregson Associates, Beccles, Suffolk
Printed and bound in Spain

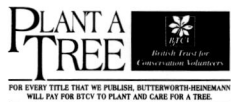

Contents

Section A
Basic principles

Patient assessment

Preoperative assessment

Before attempting any form of corneal surgery it is essential to assess the patient fully, including an assessment of the patient's (or his family's) expectations of surgery, and his intellectual and physical ability to look after his eye. For example, patients who are unable to recognize the symptoms of rejection or infection in a graft may be more exposed to sight-threatening problems than if they had not undergone surgery.

LOCAL FACTORS

The ocular environment must be as healthy as possible and elective surgery should be delayed until this is so. The lids should be in the normal anatomical position with a normal range of movement. Defects, such as entropion or lid notches, should be corrected. The margins should be clean and free from infection. Blepharitis may lead to endophthalmitis if this precaution is missed (Fig. 1.1). A clean, healthy and plentiful tear film is ideal, but a dry eye is not an absolute contraindication to surgery. Every effort should be made to ameliorate the tear film, including both the use of tear substitutes (without preservatives, in some instances, if frequent use is necessary) and

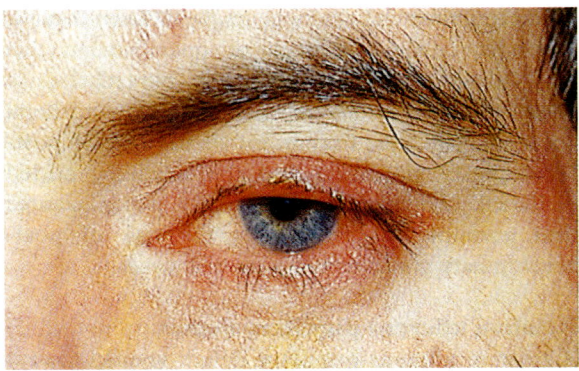

Fig. 1.1.

punctal occlusion in appropriate cases. If an emergency procedure is required, attention has to be given to this problem postoperatively.

Lacrimal drainage obstruction should also be cleared before ocular surgery, since a mucocoele is a potent source of bacteria.

Conjunctival scarring should be noted. Severe trachomatous scarring or pemphigoid will not lead to a successful graft because the metaplastic limbal conjunctival cells will not permit migration of healthy epithelial cells across the new graft. Loss of conjunctival goblet cells leads to tear-film instability and delayed healing.

Prior to undertaking refractive surgery, we would now recommend that the cornea be assessed by videokeratoscopy. This may provide valuable information which is not so obvious by other forms of assessment.

INTRINSIC FACTORS

The presence of a long-standing squint should always be sought, since this may indicate underlying amblyopia. It might also give rise to postoperative diplopia, which can be difficult to control.

Intraocular pressure

Before undertaking any graft, one must ensure that the patient is not suffering from uncontrolled glaucoma. Any existing glaucoma should be under excellent control because corneal grafting will exacerbate the problem. Uncontrolled glaucoma, or an intraocular pressure only controlled on maximum tolerated medical therapy, is an indication for trabeculectomy 3 months before undertaking keratoplasty. The presence of a failed trabeculectomy may suggest the need for silicone drainage tubing and keratoplasty. Alternatively and possibly preferably, consideration may be given to combined drainage surgery and keratoplasty. In this circumstance, almost certainly the use of mitomycin C will be necessary to maintain a functioning bleb.

In normotensive eyes, an attempt should be made to assess the drainage angle. Where there is extensive corneal oedema or opacification this may prove difficult, but it is nevertheless a valuable exercise. More than 90° of peripheral anterior synechiae may point to the risk of postkeratoplasty glaucoma and the need for added vigilance. There is unfortunately no guarantee that gonioplasty can reduce the risk of postkeratoplasty glaucoma in high-risk cases.

Relative afferent pupillary defect

A relative afferent pupillary defect should always be sought. It is disappointing for both patient and surgeon to find a clear graft with a detached retina or atrophic optic nerve behind it. An ultrasound scan may be helpful.

The lens

The lens should also be carefully assessed. Any significant cataract will increase after a graft, due partly to the increased inflammation and change in aqueous dynamics, and partly to the use of long-term topical steroids. Cataract may be removed extracapsularly and a posterior chamber lens inserted at the time of keratoplasty. This combined procedure is not only safer than two separate operations, but offers quicker visual rehabilitation for the patient. The question of biometry is difficult, since the lens power calculation depends on both the axial length and the average keratometry. In larger units, where this surgery is common, the surgeon may be able to produce a nomogram to approximate to his usual postoperative keratometry but in most cases only educated guesses are possible as to the likely average Ks. Nevertheless, biometry helps to avoid surprises with abnormally shaped eyes.

In eyes that are already aphakic or pseudophakic the presence of vitreous in the anterior chamber should be identified. Such eyes will require anterior vitrectomy. Consideration should also be given at this time to planning whether a secondary lens implant or lens exchange will be required.

DONOR MATERIAL

Many surgeons consider that the use of tissue-matched donor material enhances the prognosis for graft survival in penetrating keratoplasty. The question then arises as to how many mismatches may be acceptable; up to three are taken as the maximum, but at this level there can be very little advantage over random assignment. The more matches required, the longer the patient can expect to wait for a suitable donor, and in some cases the delay in surgery may not be justifiable. Current research may answer some of these questions but so far the reports are confused and not conclusive.

PROGNOSIS

Part of the work-up of the patient should include the ability to answer questions about prognosis for corneal surgery. For keratoplasty, the obvious question concerns the chance of the graft remaining clear. The

5-year survival for grafts in our unit experience varies from 99% in first grafts in eyes with keratoconus, through about 90% in Fuchs' dystrophy, to 65% for herpes simplex keratitis or pseudophakic bullous keratopathy and about 50% for grafts in perforated infected corneas. A less obvious, but nonetheless important question is the time it may take for the patient to reach a useful level of acuity (e.g. 6/12) through the graft with any necessary refractive correction. For keratoconus, the cumulative time for 90% of patients to reach this level may be as long as 3 years. Much of this time is accounted for by the 15–20% of patients who will be offered astigmatic correction by graft refractive surgery (see Ch. 20). This latter procedure is in itself unpredictable but following it 90% of patients are using 6/12 vision within 6 months.

REJECTION

Patients undergoing penetrating keratoplasty must also be warned of the possibility of graft rejection. Even in quiet eyes, such as keratoconus, as many as 20% of patients will experience a rejection episode, but nearly all of these are reversible with appropriate treatment. In emergency grafts this figure may rise to over 80%, with as many as one-third failing directly as a result of a rejection episode. Patients whose eyes are aphakic or have poor, as yet uncorrected, acuity may be less able to appreciate some of the early symptoms of rejection and present later for treatment.

In cases of elective surgery for the correction of simple errors of refraction, such as radial keratotomy, a patient's expectation will be very different. Such patients already have good corrected vision and expect this to be maintained. They also wish to know how predictable the surgery will be – in the case of radial keratotomy there is a 70% chance of being within 1 dioptre of the desired endpoint. Epikeratophakia is a good deal less accurate than this. As yet the authors have no data for excimer laser. For low myopia, (6 dioptres and astigmatism of not more than 2 dioptres) excimer laser offers a good refractive correction. For more extreme errors excimer laser techniques remain experimental and unproven.

Standard preoperative preparation

Whether the operation will be performed under local or general anaesthesia, the operation site will need to be prepared for surgery. It is no longer necessary to cut eyelashes but the lid margins should be clean and free from infection (see above). Topical chloramphenicol drops four times a day for 24 hours before surgery may be used. At the time of the block or as soon as the patient is on the operating table, if under general anaesthesia, a few drops of 5% povidone iodine in aqueous solution should be instilled into the conjunctival sac. The same solution should be used to paint the skin around the eye, dried off and the plastic drape applied. Care should be taken to have the eyelashes covered by the drapes.

2

Videokeratoscopy

Detailed discussion of all aspects of videokeratoscopy (VKS) requires a book in itself. Some aspects of its usage may, however, be useful to the reader.

For many years anterior segment surgeons have used Purkinje's first image to assess corneal shape and its changes. The placido disc and Keiler keratoscope still provide useful information at a fraction of the cost of a videokeratoscope. The videokeratoscope uses the same principles. It differs in as much as numerical analyses are performed on several thousand points on the captured video image. The algorithms that are employed to do this are not usually published and to an extent the observer is dependent upon the mathematical skills of the programmer as much as his own skill in capturing the best image. This becomes important when dealing with corneas which vary significantly from the norm, e.g. severely ectatic corneas. Absolute values of dioptric power may differ from one device to another but sequential change should be reasonably valid provided the devices are calibrated regularly. It is important to bear in mind that the colour picture produced by most devices is not an exaggerated photographic representation of the shape of the cornea but is a map of the cornea. It should also be remembered that the image actually represents the surface of the tear film rather than the cornea and this too can give rise to anomalies.

It is advisable to capture the video image prior to other examinations, particularly tonometry or use of a diagnostic contact lens which can imprint on the surface epithelium and distort the tear film, leading to poor quality images or inaccuracies.

Whether the expense of a videokeratoscope can be justified is debatable and the authors take the view that it is a desirable extra rather than a sine qua non for the average unit. There are exceptions, however, and present best practice guidelines for excimer laser refractive surgery would appear to insist upon the use of a VKS as part of the routine pre-assessment and postoperative monitoring of the cornea.

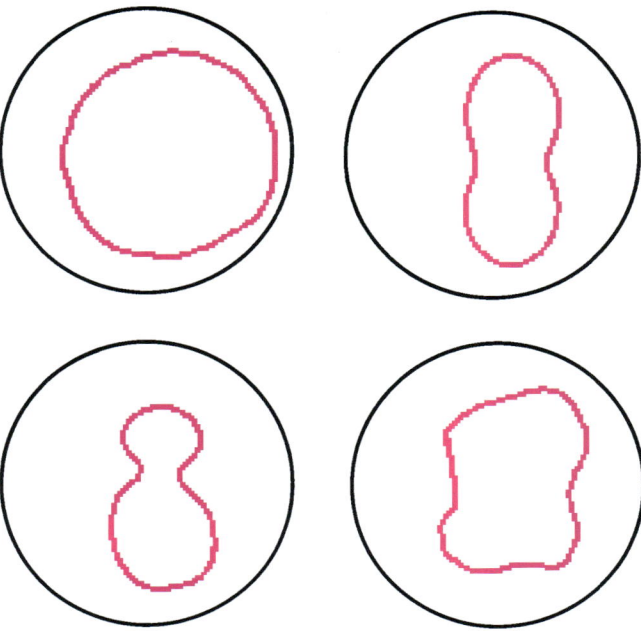

Fig. 2.1.

NORMAL PATTERNS

Initially a small number of standard patterns were described to cover the vast majority of corneas but as we gain more experience more complex categorizations are being described (Fig. 2.1).

The normal pattern appears to be of a flatter pattern temporally or of a regular astigmatism which may be demonstrated by a bowtie appearance which may be symmetric or asymmetric (Fig. 2.2); or a more irregular pattern may also be normal.

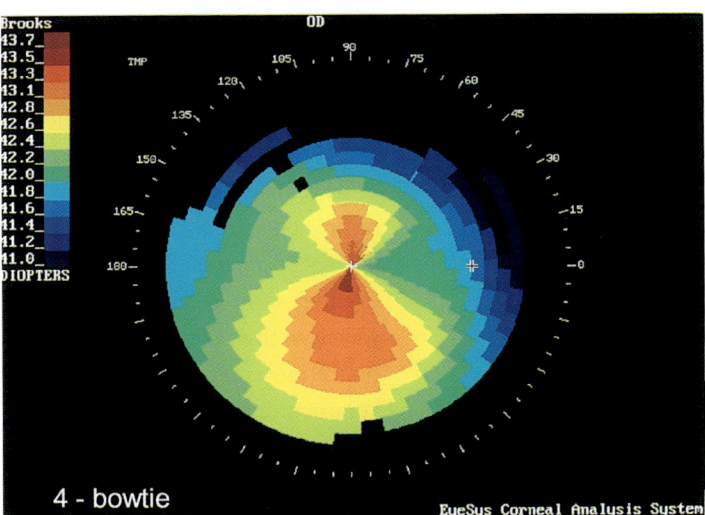

Fig. 2.2.

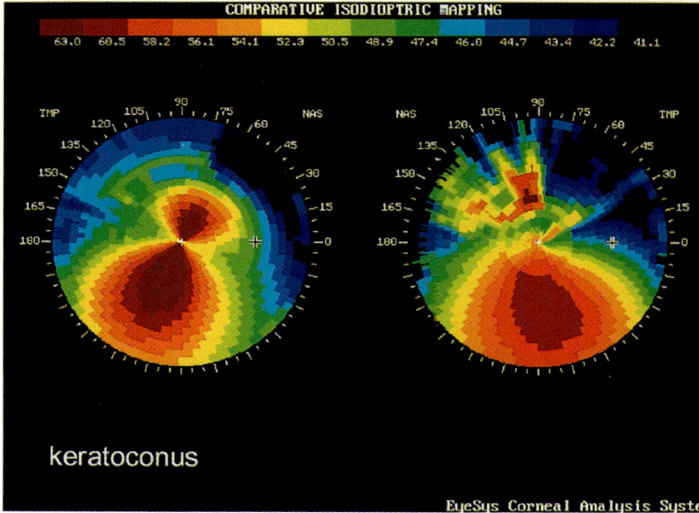

Fig. 2.3.

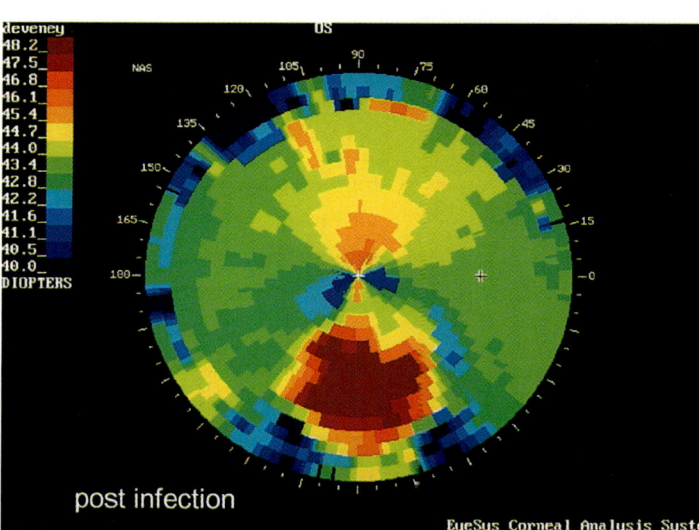

Fig. 2.4.

Keratoconus can be identified by the eccentric steep ectasia below the optic axis (Fig. 2.3). The keratoscope is sensitive in identifying keratoconus which is why many people advocate its use prior to excimer laser BUT the authors would emphasize that it is not more sensitive than the oil drop appearance on ophthalmoscopy (or scissoring on retinoscopy) which is believed to be the most sensitive test of keratoconus.

Corneal distortion as a result of trauma or infection can also be highlighted and can help suggest when a contact lens may be useful in the management of these situations (Fig 2.4).

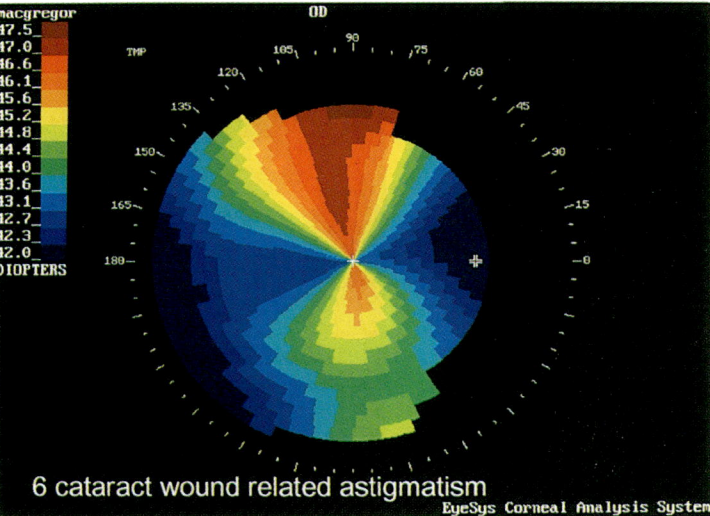

Fig. 2.5.

POSTOPERATIVE ASTIGMATISM

Where VKS becomes more helpful is in the assessment and monitoring of refractive changes in the cornea. It should be remembered that the cornea is elastic and changes in one meridian may have effects in another. The isodioptric map will indicate the degree of astigmatism and its axis but care may be required in interpreting this and estimating possible interventive surgery. Figure 2.5, for example, demonstrates an asymmetric astigmatism and may suggest that the problem is related to the upper right-hand quadrant of the patient's eye. Knowing that this is a postoperative cataract wound supports this and reviewing the video image (Fig. 2.6) reveals that the rings are indeed distorted in the appropriate quadrant. Removal of sutures (which would be too tight) or

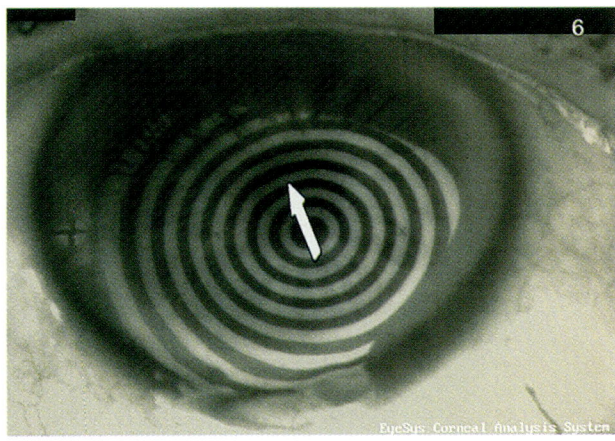

Fig. 2.6.

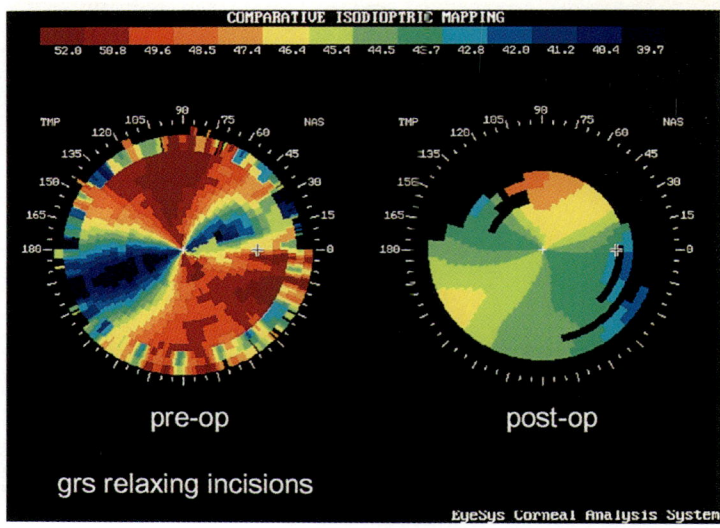

Fig. 2.7.

revision of the wound which may be overriding would be indicated depending upon the circumstances.

Astigmatism is, however, more common after keratoplasty. Figure 2.7 shows the preoperative appearance of a graft with sutures removed which had intolerable astigmatism despite a relatively cylindrical error. This was satisfactorily corrected by relieving incisions (as described in Chapter 19) which is readily demonstrated by VKS. Again the isodioptric map needs to be reviewed in conjunction with the refraction and keratoscopic image before deciding upon the appropriate technique and position of incisions.

Figure 2.8 shows the preoperative appearance and the results of

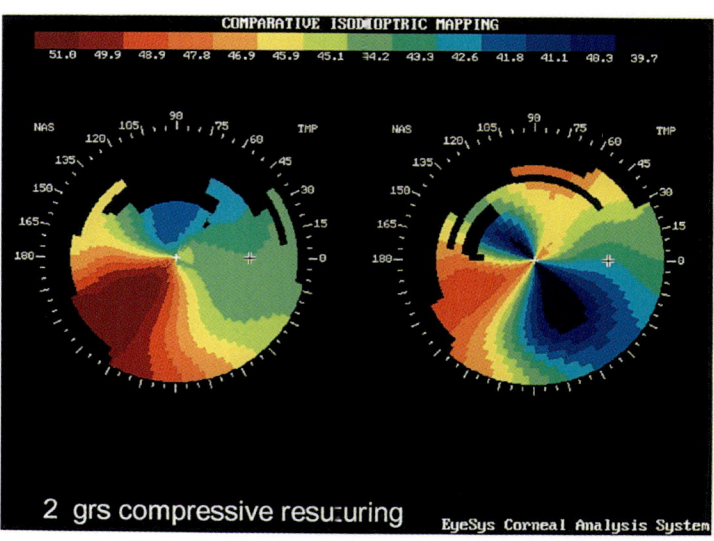

Fig. 2.8.

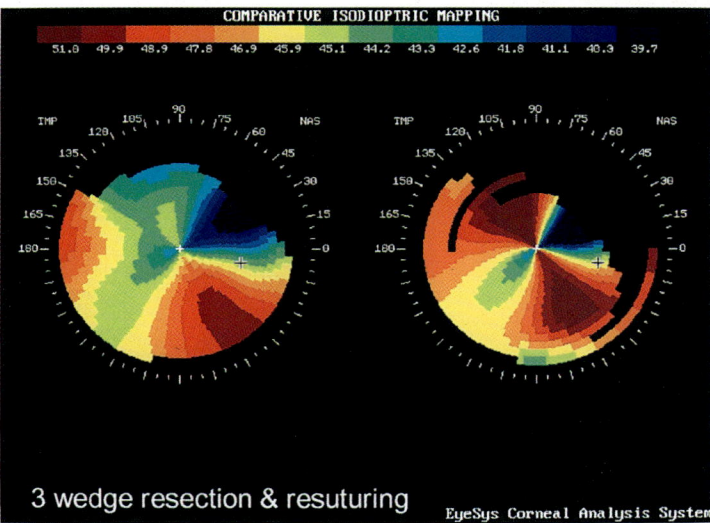

Fig. 2.9.

compressive resuturing after removal of all sutures more than 15 months after the graft refractive surgery. The eye is still astigmatic but more symmetric in pattern, and it is now at a tolerable level. Selective suture removal may be monitored by this technique and for interim short-term results may give a quicker evaluation than subjective refraction.

Figure 2.9 shows the results of a wedge resection and resuturing (not described herein) for an unusual case where, in a perforation, an excessively oversized button had been used. Marked anisekonia followed with 12 dioptres (spherical equivalent of myopia). A contact lens could not be tolerated and there was additional astigmatism. Wedge resection reduced the myopia to tolerable limits and although not eliminated the degree of astigmatism was also tolerated and the patient was visually rehabilitated. The technique of wedge resection is indicated so infrequently and can be so unpredictable that the authors have not included it in the sections on surgical techniques.

One of the most useful aspects of VKS had been the help it has given in understanding the optical results of some corneal grafts. One is occasionally faced with a graft that appears clear but yet subjective refraction fails to improve the vision to a level which approximates the pinhole acuity. VKS often reveals that such grafts have a much more complex shape than might have been suspected. Figure 2.10 demonstrates such an appearance which suggests 'warping' of the graft. This is often not relieved by removal of the odd suture. Instead removal of all

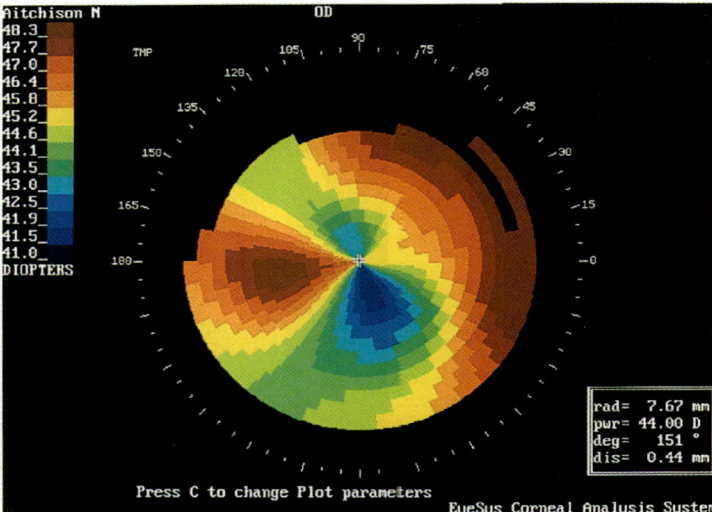

Fig. 2.10.

sutures may be necessary possibly combined with wound revision and resuturing.

REFRACTIVE SURGERY

The effect on corneal shape of other forms of refractive surgery can be readily demonstrated by VKS. Figure 2.11 shows the central flattening

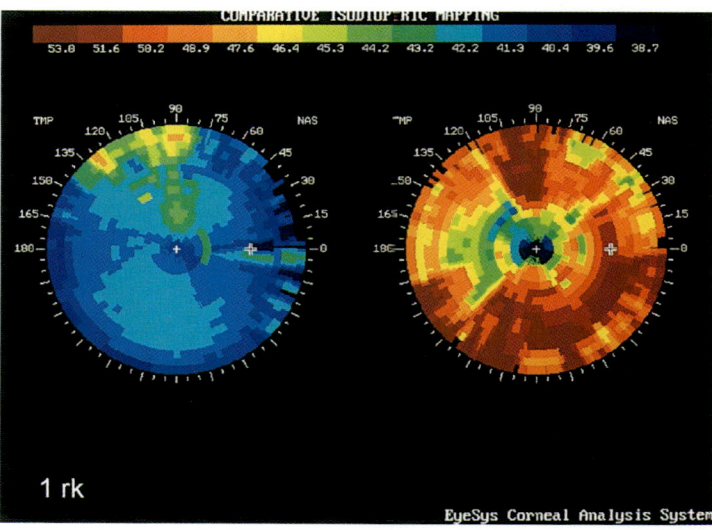

Fig. 2.11.

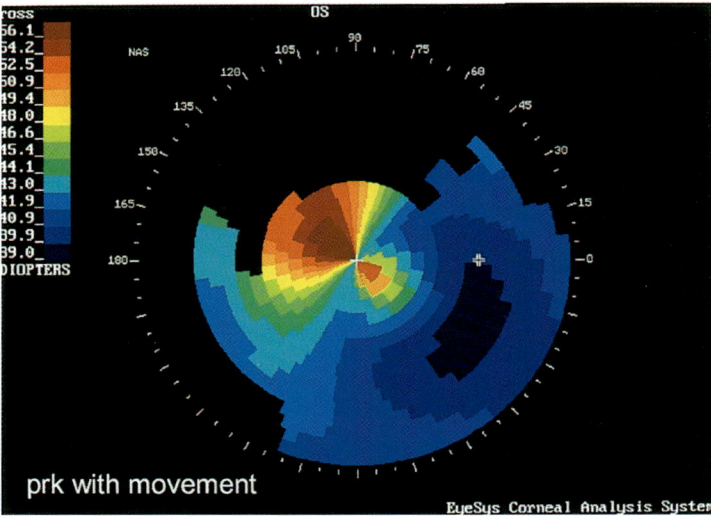

Fig. 2.12.

produced by radial keratotomy. The videoscopic appearances are remarkably similar to those changes produced by excimer laser.

The changes can of course be monitored with time and stabilization of the healing process documented. Any inaccuracy of the laser cut can be highlighted. Figure 2.12 shows an excimer laser photorefractive keratectomy (PRK) which was complicated by movement of the patient's eye during treatment. This has resulted in a very uneven profile producing an irregular astigmatism which has proved difficult to correct.

SUMMARY

The advent of this technique has been a substantial benefit to the assessment of corneal disorders both pre- and postoperatively.

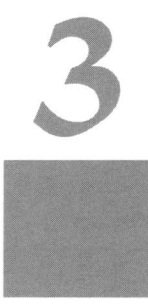

3

Instruments for corneal microsurgery

Basic instruments

For accurate and atraumatic surgery upon the cornea, instruments need to be selected with care. We would suggest that a basic set would include the following:

1. Speculum of light wire construction either of the Pierse or Barraquer design.
2. Tissue holding forceps:
   a. with fine jaws and notched tips
   b. very fine toothed forceps, straight or of Collibri design
   c. Collibri toothed forceps
   d. tissue fixation forceps (two pairs Jayle's or Lister's).
3. Suture typing forceps (two pairs). These should be short with fine plain ends, preferably of titanium with tungsten coating to provide a very strong gripping surface.
4. Needle holders, also fine ended, preferably of titanium with a *straight* tip and tungsten coating of the gripping surface.
5. Scissors:
   a. right- and left-cutting, narrow-bladed, curved corneal scissors
   b. fine, long, narrow-bladed, straight and angled scissors for intracameral use (capsule, iris, fibrous bands, etc.)
   c. suture-cutting scissors (Westcott design). Also used for preparation of conjunctival flaps.
6. Fine-tipped bipolar cautery with variable control.
7. Fine, smooth-edge iris repositor.
8. Knives:
   a. straight-edged or trifaceted diamond
   b. disposable fine-tipped steel blades with a suitable blade holder.

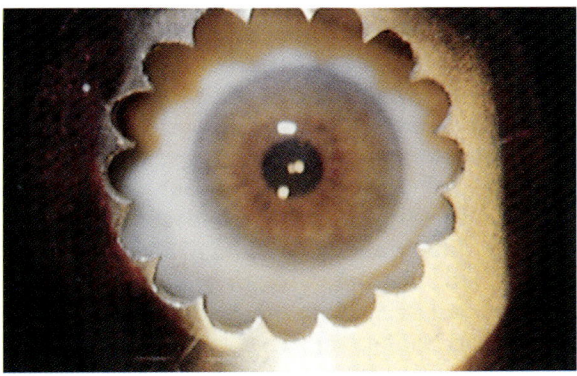

Fig. 3.1.

9. Trephines:

   a. a range of ultrasharp, disposable blades for preparing donor buttons by a punching technique

   b. a range of re-usable hollow trephines of the following sizes in millimetres: 2, 4, 5, 5.5, 6, 6.5, 7, 7.5, 7.75, 8.0, 8.25, 8.5, 9.0, 10.0, 11.0 and 12.0. Only those sizes in the centre of the range are used frequently.

10. A donor eye stand. The authors recommend the stand designed by Pierse and Steele, which allows for variable control of the intraocular pressure (Fig. 3.1; see also Figs 7.1).

11. Punching blocks of silicone or similar material for donor disc punching.

12. Sutures and needles:

   a. 5 or 6/0 silk or braided nylon on a cutting-edged needle for rectus sutures

   b. 7/0 silk on a cutting-edged needle for corneal overlay sutures

   c. 8/0 or 7/0 vicryl of 8/0 virgin silk on 6-mm spatulate needle for scleral and conjunctival suturing

   d. 9/0 and 10/0 nylon on 6-mm curved spatulate needles for corneal suturing

   e. 10/0 prolene on 8-mm taper-cut needles for uveal tissue repair

   f. 10/0 and 11/0 mersilene for graft refractive surgery.

13. Cannulae: 30 gauge, lacrimal and Southampton cannulae are all useful for corneal surgery, together with a variety of syringes – 2, 5 and 10 ml capacity.

14. Visco-elastic material either as sodium hyaluronate or 2% hydroxypropylmethyl-cellulose.

15. For suture removal, fine-tipped, plain forceps are useful. We particularly like the Rice forceps design which has a carved tip.

Wherever possible the authors recommend the use of small titanium instruments for microsurgery. These have the advantages of being light and strong, rustproof and non-magnetic, and having matt-finish, non-reflecting surfaces.

Special instruments

Keratometer

All corneal surgery is capable of altering corneal curvature and perioperative keratometry is sometimes recommended to improve the surgeon's control of this factor. However, surgical keratometers attached to the surgical microscope are very expensive indeed, and the authors are doubtful whether the cost can be justified. Qualitative keratometry can always be achieved perioperatively by the use of a safety pin with a circular end, which may be held a short distance above the cornea so as to produce a circular or oval reflection on the corneal surface, easily visible through the microscope. This simple device is surprisingly sensitive.

An alternative, if slightly more expensive, instrument is the Maloney keratosope, which resembles a hollow truncated cone with graded width grooves on the internal surface. For accuracy of use, the intraocular pressure should be normal and the eye must not be distorted. When the keratometer is held on the cornea a series of concentric circles are seen reflected on the cornea. Any distortion is immediately apparent. We feel that though this is a useful technique at the end of graft surgery it is not necessarily very reliable whereas in graft refractive surgery the keratoscope is much more useful.

Aspiration/irrigation equipment

Aspiration/irrigation equipment is required for the satisfactory removal of cortical material during extracapsular cataract extraction. Cannulae of the type described by McIntyre or Simco are both suitable for this procedure, and are also recommended for open sky aspiration/irrigation. An automated system is slightly less easy to control.

Surgical microscope

A surgical microscope is an essential piece of equipment for the modern corneal surgeon. The magnification it provides is essential for accuracy of wound control and for the avoidance of peroperative complications which can otherwise escape attention. A wide variety of surgical microscopes are available, but that chosen should provide a comfortable working distance between the objective lens and the surface of the eye, as wide a surgical field as possible, a good depth of focus, variable magnification, and illumination which should include both co-axial and non-co-axial light beams. In addition, the surgical microscope should be fitted with an attachment for the use of the surgical assistant, the assistant's view being as close as possible to that of the surgeon and fully binocular. An assistant's microscope fitted to a beam splitter is less than ideal, as it eliminates all stereopsis. Ideally, it should also be possible to fit the surgical microscope with both video and photographic equipment.

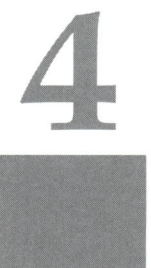

4

Microsurgical techniques, including corneal wound repair

Microsurgical techniques for the cornea are principally concerned with the making and repair of corneal wounds. Lamellar dissection will be discussed in a later chapter (see Chapter 17).

Incisions

These may be straight or curved:

Straight incisions (Fig. 4.1) (e.g. as for radial keratotomy)
Straight incisions are best made with a diamond knife or very sharp steel blade, and using a toothed limbal fixation forceps to secure the

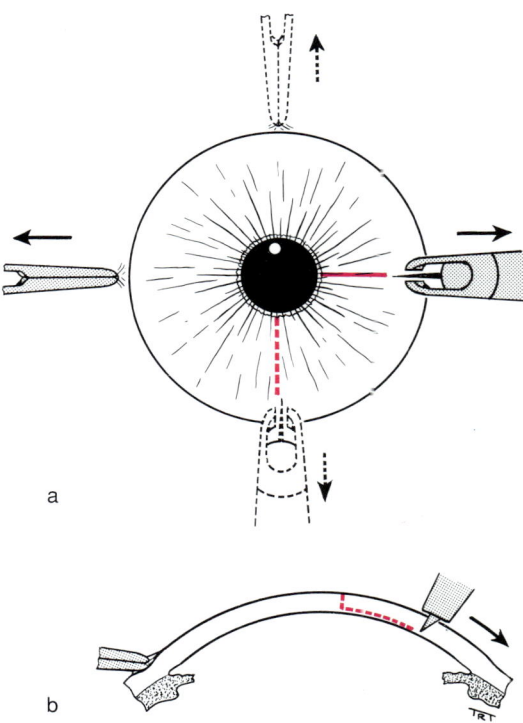

a

b

Fig. 4.1.

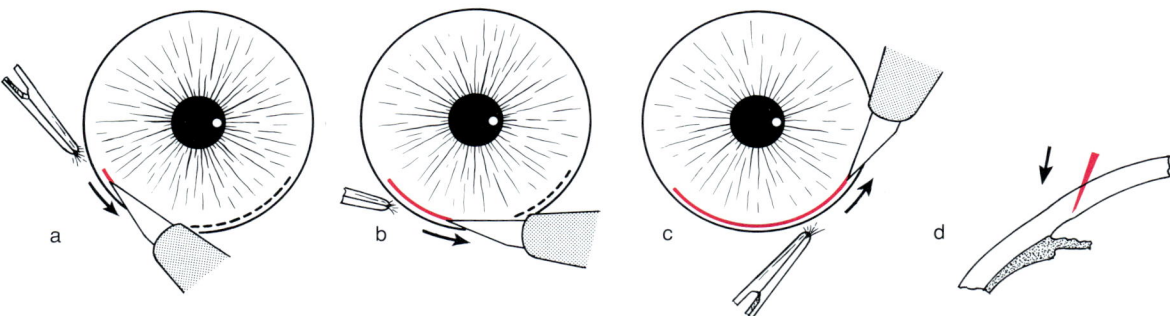

Fig. 4.2.

globe and to provide the necessary countertraction to the passage of the knife through the corneal tissue. This countertraction should always be as close as possible to the line of cut made by the knife so that the knife will move smoothly and in a straight line. The alignment of the forceps and the direction of incision also minimizes the tendency for the eye to rotate upon its anteroposterior axis. Most corneal incisions are made normal to the corneal surface. The important exception to this rule is the corneal incision for extracapsular cataract surgery which is classically back-sloping so as to form a leak-resistant corneal valve effect.

Curved incisions (Fig. 4.2)
Where a curved incision is required (e.g. cataract wound or peripheral lamellar bed preparation), the fixation forceps are used to grasp the limbus as close as possible to the incision's commencement. The forceps are then transferred to the lip of the wound and progressively advanced along the curvature behind the knife as the incision proceeds. This improves the accuracy of the cut by ensuring that the countertraction provided by the forceps is always in the line of the incision (Fig. 4.2). For the curved edge of a peripheral lamellar bed, the curvature is best marked out on the epithelium with the edge of an appropriately sized trephine, usually of large diameter. The knife can then be used to follow the indent so produced, using the fixation forceps in the same manner as described above.

Corneal wound closure (Fig. 4.3; this specifically does not refer to keratoplasty wounds)

Corneal wounds are best closed using 10/0 nylon suture material mounted on a 6-mm curved spatulate needle. These needles are supremely sharp and it requires little effort in tissue fixation to pass a

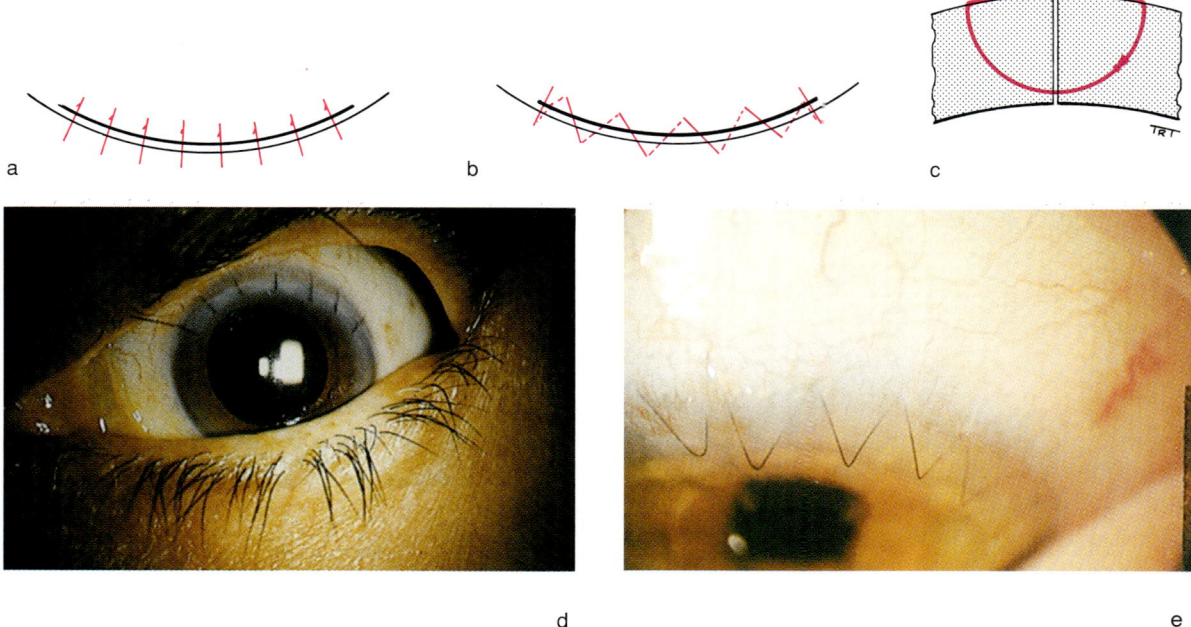

Fig. 4.3.

needle through the tough corneal stroma. Care must be taken never to allow the tip of the needle to touch the fixation forceps, the needle holder or any other metallic object, as this will immediately damage the needle tip and impair its sharpness. This in turn leads to a significant increase in the force required to pass the needle through the tissue, causing tissue distortion and endothelial damage.

All corneal sutures affect the corneal curvature, so care must be taken to avoid distortion which can lead to high degrees of astigmatic error. Suture bites should therefore always be deep (to obtain full depth of wound closure) and short (to minimize unwanted distortional forces). The tension in the suture is designed to make the corneal wound leak-free only, and must not be over-tightened. Ends of nylon must be cut as close as possible to the knot, which must then always be turned into the suture track to avoid surface irritation. Some knots, e.g. during corneal grafting, can conveniently be tied in the wound itself.

Corneal wound sutures may be either interrupted or continuous. Interrupted sutures are always placed perpendicular to the wound to avoid wound distortion. Continuous sutures in a long straight or curved wound must also be inserted so as to avoid the introduction of rotational torque. In order to achieve this, a single running suture must be placed across the wound at an angle, while a double running

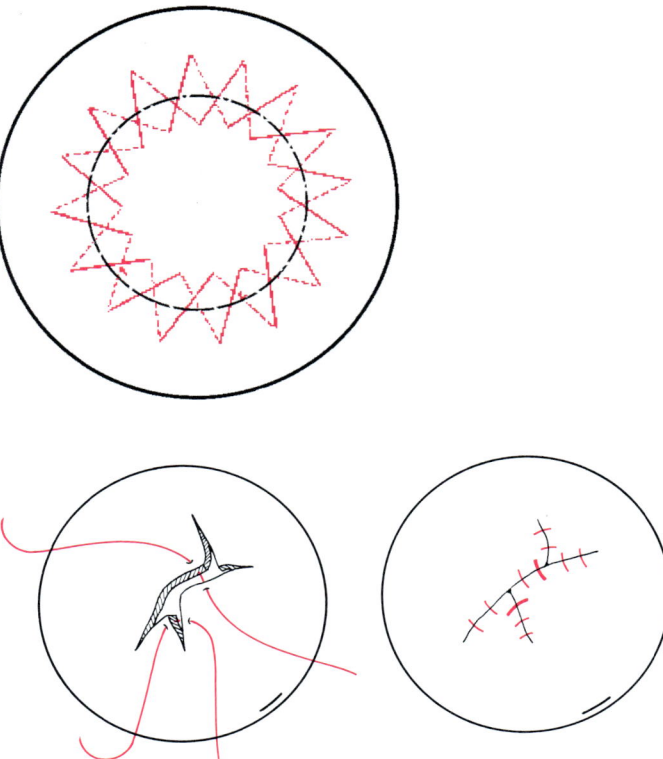

Fig. 4.4.

Fig. 4.5.

suture may have the bites introduced perpendicular to the wound. The torque forces in one direction are thus balanced by similar torque forces in the other direction (Fig. 4.3). In principle, however, the authors are not in favour of the so-called bootlace suture which has overlapping sutures exposed on the ocular surface (Fig. 4.4). The area of crossover may attract mucus and infection.

When suturing an irregular traumatic wound (Figs 4.5 and 4.6) it is always preferable first to make a peripheral paracentesis through which the anterior chamber may be deepened as required as the repair proceeds. The use of visco-elastic material greatly facilitates this process.

Occasionally it may be necessary to insert a 'purse-string' type suture into stellate lacerations. This should start in the wound and be placed at a distance at least half the length of a normal suture bite behind the apex of the wound. The suture should be at mid-stromal depth. Each apex should be sutured in turn until the full 360° has been sutured. The tension can be adjusted until the wound is water tight and not overly compressed and the knot completed. With some irregular wounds it

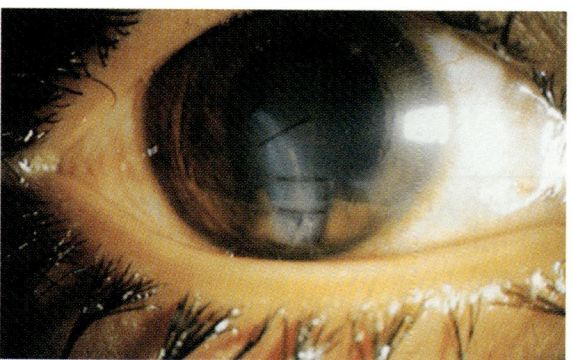

Fig. 4.6.

may not be possible to achieve a watertight closure due to loss of tissue, or distortion. Tight sutures should be readjusted or replaced, slack ones tightened or replaced. If the wound continues to leak it may be possible to seal it by the application of cyanoacrylate glue (see Ch. 18). It is preferable to do this than to consider a keratoplasty in the acute situation when the eye is severely inflamed and contused.

In this book on corneal surgery we felt it inappropriate to discuss phacoemulsification and sutures (self-sealing wounds) for cataract surgery. We are aware that many of the incisions are sited in the cornea, and that they will have an influence on corneal topography resulting in mild flattening of the axis of astigmatism of approximately 0.5 dioptres.

Anaesthesia for corneal surgery

Many superficial corneal procedures may be satisfactorily performed under topical anaesthesia alone. In very anxious individuals this may be supplemented with sedation, administered either orally or intravenously. If for some reason the patient is unable to cooperate or there is a significant risk of corneal perforation during the procedure, general anaesthesia is a much better option. Ocular akinesis and control of intraocular pressure can be readily provided. In selected patients, however, a local anaesthetic block can also provide good operating conditions. Traditionally this has been a retrobulbar block with a facial nerve block, both administered by the surgeon. On occasion, serious surgical complications such as globe perforation or retrobulbar haemorrhage have occurred and there has been a move towards alternative techniques. The recognition also, of occasional systemic complications of ophthalmic local blocks, especially in medically compromised patients, has led to the involvement of the anaesthetist with patients undergoing procedures under local block. The Joint Working Party report on Anaesthesia in Ophthalmic Surgery recommends that the anaesthetist should be involved in the choice of anaesthetic, the preparation and counselling of the patient, performance of the block, monitoring during the procedure and the treatment of any complications.

With economic pressures dictating an increase in day-case surgery, there is pressure to perform many types of corneal surgery on a day-care basis. These operations may be performed under local or general anaesthesia, but adequate arrangements must be made for ophthalmic follow-up and for home care.

General anaesthesia

Indications

1. Patient preference.
2. Surgical preference.

3. Patients who would be unable to cooperate in lying flat and still on an operating table. This includes the very young, the confused, the very deaf, patients who do not understand the language, patients with uncontrollable cough and patients with uncontrolled movement, such as the tremor of Parkinson's disease.

Contraindications

1. Airway difficulties, such as a known or suspected difficult intubation.
2. Respiratory failure in end-stage obstructive airways disease, or musculoskeletal diseases.
3. Cardiac failure in severe ischaemic heart disease or cardiac arrhythmias.
4. Adverse reaction to anaesthetic agents. This may be inherited as in malignant hyperthermia or due to allergy.

Preoperative assessment

All of the following should be performed at the booking clinic.

1. Full medical history and examination, including weight and blood pressure measurement.
2. Haemoglobin estimation in patients with signs or symptoms of anaemia.
3. Sickle-cell testing if sickle disease indicated from racial origin or history.
4. Urea and electrolyte estimation in patients taking diuretics, those with signs or symptoms of renal disease or with diabetes.
5. Blood sugar estimation in diabetics.
6. Urinalysis in all patients.
7. Electrocardiogram in patients with signs and symptoms of cardiac disease or myocardial ischaemia, those with systemic disease known to be associated with cardiac problems (hypertension, diabetes, etc.), or in all patients over 60 years of age.
8. Chest X-ray if indicated by signs and symptoms.

If necessary, patients must be referred to the physician for the best control of their medical conditions and to the physiotherapist for the best control of chronic obstructive airways disease.

Techniques

Although corneal surgery does not usually cause much surgical stimulation, any technique used must guarantee ocular akinesis and reliable control of intraocular pressure if the eye is opened.

Premedication

Patients are starved for 6 hours. A suitable premedication would consist of a mild anxiolytic such as oral temazepam 0.3 mg/kg one hour preoperatively in combination with an antiemetic such as metaclopramide 10 mg orally. In cases of hiatus hernia or oesophageal reflux an H_2 blocker such as ranitidine 150 mg orally would be given in addition.

Induction of anaesthesia

The aims of induction of general anaesthesia for ophthalmic surgery are to secure the airway and to prevent any rise in intraocular pressure due to coughing or straining. The use of the induction agent propofol 1–2 mg/kg with a potent short-acting opiate such as alfentanil 10 μg/kg with or without the muscle relaxant vecuronium 0.1 mg/kg provides excellent conditions in most patients. In elderly or frail patients care must be taken that this technique does not drop the blood pressure or pulse rate too low. The airway may be satisfactorily secured using the laryngeal mask airway which avoids the laryngeal stimulation of intubation. In very obese patients, those with increased pulmonary compliance or with symptomatic oesophageal reflux the airway is best secured by an endotracheal tube.

Maintenance

In superficial corneal surgery satisfactory operating conditions can be achieved by allowing the patient to breath spontaneously with an inhalational anaesthetic. However, if central eye position is vital, if there is a high risk of corneal perforation or if the eye is to be open during surgery, the best operating conditions are provided by paralysis and hyperventilation. Hypnosis may be maintained with an inhalational agent or with a propofol infusion either by a manually operated infusion pump (TIVA) or by Target controlled infusion (TCI). Propofol infusions are relatively expensive but have the advantage of rapid recovery from anaesthesia without 'hangover' and reduced nausea and vomiting.

Reversal and extubation

The patient should emerge smoothly from anaesthesia, without coughing or straining. Careful attention must be paid to airway maintenance and removal of secretions. The laryngeal mask airway is a very reliable way of obtaining these conditions as the patient will tolerate it without coughing until fully awake when they simply spit it out. Postoperative nausea and vomiting is not usually a problem following corneal surgery, but if the patient has a strong history, prophylaxis with droperidol (a dopaminergic antagonist) in a dose of 2.5–5.0 mg intravenously during surgery may be of help.

Monitoring

The patient should be monitored in accordance with the published recommendations of the Association of Anaesthetists. Monitoring should start prior to induction of anaesthesia and continue into the recovery period. The following would be considered essential during corneal surgery:

1. Presence of the anaesthetist throughout the anaesthetic.
2. Pulse oximeter.
3. Electrocardiograph.
4. Indirect blood pressure measurement.
5. Capnograph.
6. Peripheral nerve stimulator in paralysed patients.
7. Anaesthetic machine monitors such as an oxygen analyser or ventilator disconnect alarm.
8. The ability to measure core body temperature if the need arose, although it is not routinely monitored in adult corneal surgery.

Complications

Serious complications are rare. Intubation difficulties, laryngeal spasm following extubation and respiratory depression postoperatively are some of the most serious. Damage to teeth can endanger the airway and certainly provide medicolegal difficulties. Cardiac arrhythmias and labile blood pressures can sometimes be a problem. Minor morbidity of sore throat, headache, nausea and vomiting and sleepiness are common if care is not taken to minimize them.

Local anaesthesia

Indications

1. Patient preference.
2. Relative or absolute contraindication to general anaesthesia.

3. Uncomplicated corneal surgery of short duration, especially superficial procedures.

Contraindications

1. Patients who are unable to cooperate in lying flat and still on the operating table.
2. Allergy to local anaesthetic agents.

Preoperative assessment

This is the same as for general anaesthesia. Many patients considered as high risk for general anaesthesia are even less suitable for local anaesthesia. These patients need a thorough preoperative work-up that allows a decision on method of anaesthesia to be made between the parties concerned, the surgeon, the anaesthetist and the patient.

METHODS

There are a variety of techniques available that may be used depending on the nature of the surgery and the cooperation of the patient. Topical anaesthesia provides good surface anaesthesia without the complications of the regional blocks but the patient retains full eye movement. The classical technique of retrobulbar block provides good akinesia and anaesthesia, but usually requires a supplemental facial nerve block to paralyse orbicularis oculi. Rare but serious complications have occurred, including retrobulbar haemorrhage, globe perforation, damage to the optic nerve or ophthalmic artery and spread of local anaesthetic to the brainstem along the optic nerve dural sheath. Peribulbar anaesthesia was introduced to avoid these complications by placing large volumes of anaesthetic solution outside the muscle cone with the needle tip no further back than the equator of the eye. The solution spreads throughout the compartments of the eye and provides delayed but very satisfactory operating conditions.

Any technique using a blindly placed sharp needle may result in serious complications including globe perforation. A more recently described technique involves the transconjunctival injection of anaesthetic solution directly into the sub-Tenon's space, in the inferonasal quadrant, using a blunt curved cannula.

Patients undergoing corneal procedures under any form of local anaesthesia still require monitoring by the anaesthetist, in case of the rare adverse reaction, to manage any complication of on-going medical conditions and to provide sedation, especially in young, fit, nervous patients. Equipment for resuscitation should be available at all times and it is recommended practice to have intravenous access in situ for the duration of the procedure.

1. Topical anaesthesia

This is commonly used for removal of sutures and small foreign bodies and in superficial surgery of the conjunctiva and cornea. The onset of corneoconjunctival anaesthesia following instillation of all the commonly used agents is within 15–20 seconds and lasts 15–20 minutes. Stinging is the main side effect and can be minimized by using a few drops of diluted anaesthetic prior to the full strength preparation. Side effects of corneal toxicity, tear-film instability and systemic effects are only a problem with prolonged use of topical anaesthetics.

Proxymetacaine HCl 0.5% (Ophthaine) produces rapid onset of superficial anaesthesia with minimal stinging. Repeated doses of one drop every 5 minutes for about five doses is required to provide deeper corneoconjunctival anaesthesia.

Oxybuprocaine HCl 0.4% (Benoxinate) also produces little stinging and little corneal toxicity.

Amethocaine HCl 0.5% and 1.0% has a slower onset time and produces more stinging than the other topical agents but provides deeper corneal anaesthesia which makes it more suitable for minor surgical procedures. It causes local hyperaemia in the eye and can be cardiotoxic in overdose.

Lignocaine HCl 4.0% is an amide-linked agent and is an over-looked topical anaesthetic for use on the eye. It is isotonic and the least toxic to the cornea of the topical anaesthetics. It produces deep anaesthesia with relatively long duration.

2. Retrobulbar anaesthesia

Retrobulbar anaesthesia, where a small volume of local anaesthetic is injected into the muscle cone behind the eye is still widely practised. A successful block provides akinesia of the extraocular muscles and anaesthesia of the eye, but in most cases the orbicularis oculi muscle has to be blocked with a facial nerve block to prevent squeezing of the eyelids.

Technique

1. Patient lies supine on a trolley with head supported on a pillow.
2. The eyes are in a neutral position.

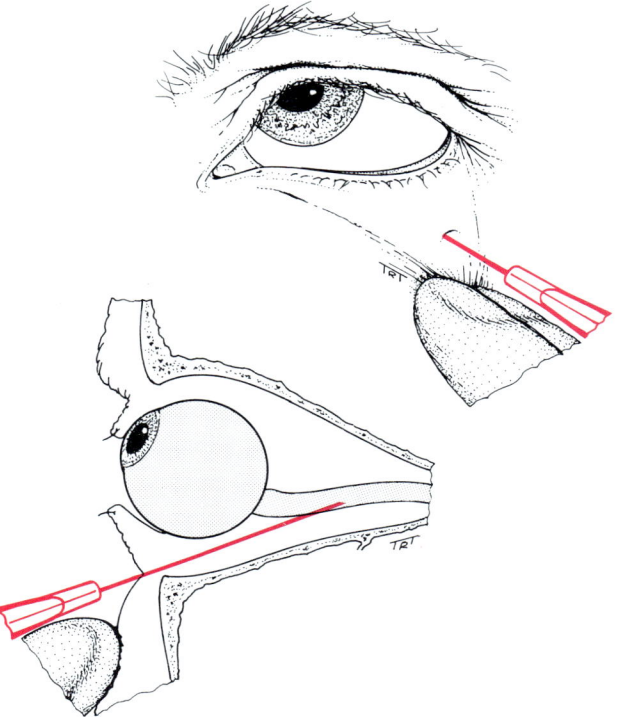

Fig. 5.1.

3. A 25 gauge 1.25 mm needle and a 5 ml syringe containing the local anaesthetic are used for the injection.

4. Standing at the level of the patient's head on the side of the eye to be blocked, the needle is inserted at the junction of the middle and outer thirds of the eye just above the infraorbital rim, at right angles to the skin. The needle is advanced until the tip lies just behind the equator of the globe. The needle direction is then re-angled in an upward and medial direction to enter the muscle cone behind the eye. Care is taken not to cross the mid-sagittal plane of the eye (Fig. 5.1).

5. Following test aspiration 3–4 ml of anaesthetic are slowly injected.

6. Ptosis of the eyelid and slight proptosis of the eye may be seen with this volume placed behind the eye.

7. The eye is closed and an oculopressor device applied for 10 minutes to produce ocular hypotony for intraocular surgery. A successful block will provide akinesia and anaesthesia within 5 minutes.

8. Pain on injection through the skin may be the most distressing part for the patient and this can be minimized by raising an intradermal bleb of 0.5% lignocaine at the needle entry site prior to the injection.

3. Peribulbar anaesthesia

First described in 1986, peribulbar anaesthesia usually consists of two injections of local anaesthetic, one inferior and one medial to the eye, the needles penetrating no further than the equator of the eye. The volume of anaesthetic used is usually enough to block the terminal branches of the facial nerve and paralyse the orbicularis oculi muscle.

Technique

1. Place the patient supine on a trolley with the head supported on a pillow.
2. The eyes are in the neutral position.
3. Stand beside the patient on the side of the eye to be blocked.
4. Anaesthetise the conjunctiva with a few drops of oxybuprocaine HCl 0.4% (Benoxinate).
5. Using a 30 gauge needle, inject about 1.0 ml of lignocaine, diluted to 0.2% with normal saline, into the outer aspect of the lower lid through the conjunctiva below the tarsal plate. This provides anaesthesia for the inferior peribulbar injection (Fig. 5.2).

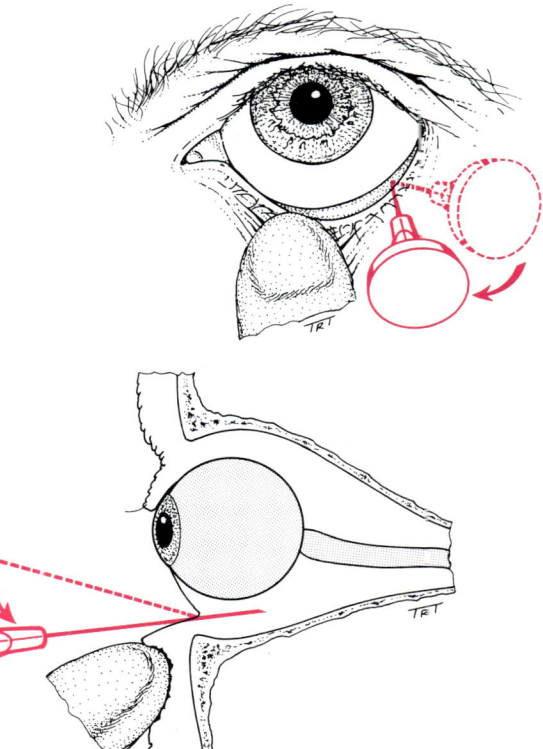

Fig. 5.2.

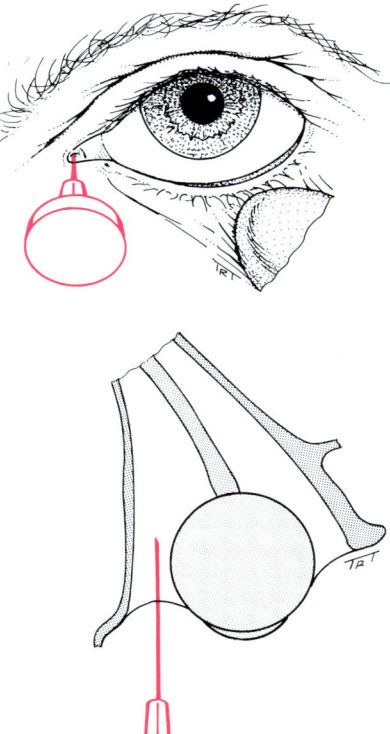

Fig. 5.3.

6. The inferotemporal injection is made using a 25 gauge 25 mm sharp needle with a 5 ml syringe containing the anaesthetic solution. The needle point is placed on the conjunctiva 2 mm out from the sclera, midway between the lateral canthus and the sagittal plane of the lateral limbus. Keeping the needle tangential to the globe, it is passed posteriorly and slightly medially to a depth of no more than 1.5 cm so that the needle tip lies in a plane sagittal to the lateral limbus (Fig. 5.2).

7. Slowly inject 2–5 ml of the anaesthetic solution, assessing intra-orbital tension digitally.

8. Maintain gentle pressure for 2 minutes. In 5% of patients this alone will give good akinesia.

9. The medial injection is given using a 25 gauge 25 mm needle with a 5 ml syringe containing the anaesthetic solution. With the needle bevel facing medially, the tip is placed medial to the medial caruncle and the needle passed posteriorly, keeping perpendicular to the face. An initial resistance may be felt at the medial check ligament, then the needle should pass without resistance to a depth of about 1.5 cm (Fig. 5.3).

10. Slowly inject 2–5 ml of the anaesthetic, digitally assessing the intraorbital tension.

11. Maintain gentle pressure for 5 minutes then assess the block. Complete ocular akinesia should be obtained without lid movement.

12. To provide suitable hypotony for intraocular surgery such as corneal graft, an oculopressor device should be employed for 10 minutes.

4. Sub-Tenon anaesthesia

This technique is usually performed by the operating surgeon just prior to surgery on the operating table. In this case topical anaesthesia should be given prior to cleaning and draping the eye to minimize patient discomfort.

Technique

1. Stand at the head of the patient.

2. If not already given, a few drops of amethocaine HCl 0.5% are applied to anaesthetise the conjunctiva.

3. With the patient looking up and outwards a small incision is made, with spring scissors, in the conjunctiva, about 5 mm from the limbus in the inferonasal quadrant of the eye.

4. Bleeding from the conjunctival vessels can be reduced by using a drop of adrenaline 0.1% on the conjunctiva prior to the incision.

5. Using a blunt, curved 19 gauge, 26 mm sub-Tenon's cannula with a 5 ml syringe containing the anaesthetic solution, a small bleb is raised at the site of the incision.

6. This allows identification and elevation of Tenon's capsule in which another small incision is made with the spring scissors.

7. Using Moorfields forceps to hold the cut conjunctival edge the cannula is inserted onto bare sclera and slid along the contour of the globe to the equator.

8. At this point 1 ml of anaesthetic solution is deposited and the cannula advanced to a total distance of about 1.5–2.0 cm depending on the size of the globe (Fig. 5.4).

9. A further 3.0–3.5 ml anaesthetic are given and the cannula withdrawn.

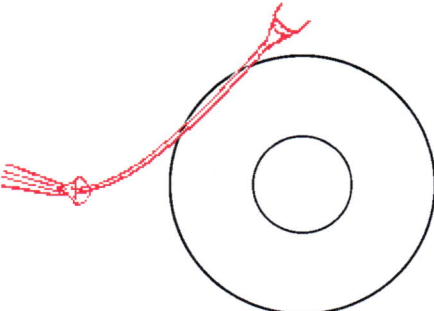

Fig. 5.4.

10. A small degree of proptosis of the globe is usually apparent at this stage.

11. In about 10 minutes there should be suitable akinesis, anaesthesia and hypotony for surgery.

THE LOCAL ANAESTHETIC MIXTURE

The characteristics of an ophthalmic block are not only determined by the technique employed but also by the local anaesthetic solution injected. The speed of onset and duration of a block, and the differential sensory to motor blockade will be affected by the particular local anaesthetic used and the volume and concentration of that anaesthetic. This can be used to tailor the anaesthetic block to the patient and to the particular surgical procedure to be undertaken.

Lignocaine HCl is usually used in a concentration of 2% for ophthalmic anaesthesia, and will produce effects within 5 minutes and provide surgical anaesthesia for 30–40 minutes.

Prilocaine HCl, again used in a concentration of 2%, will take 5–10 minutes to produce its effects but lasts for 60 minutes.

Bupivacaine HCl is used in concentrations of 0.5% and 0.75% in ophthalmic anaesthesia but is not usually used on its own but in a mixture with lignocaine. Bupivacaine has a slow onset of action on its own, up to 30 minutes onset time, and a very long duration of action of up to 4–8 hours of surgical anaesthesia.

Mixtures of equal volumes of lignocaine 2% and bupivacaine 0.5% or 0.75% are commonly used in ophthalmic blocks to provide a rapid onset and prolonged duration of the anaesthesia.

Adrenaline may be added to the local anaesthetic solution in a concentration of 5 μg/ml to increase the intensity and duration of the block. The vasoconstriction produced by the adrenaline reduces local blood flow and absorption of the anaesthetic. In some cases, where

Table 5.1. Suggested safe local anaesthetic doses

Drug	Maximum safe dose (without adrenaline) (mg/kg)	Maximum safe dose (in 70 kg person) (mg)	Volume (ml)
Lignocaine 2%	3	200	10
Prilocaine 2%	6	400	20
Bupivacaine 0.5%	2	150	30
Bupivacaine 0.75%	2	150	20

retinal blood flow is compromised, this vasoconstriction may not be desirable and a longer acting anaesthetic should be used as a means of prolonging the block.

Hyaluronidase in a dose of 5–15 IU/ml may be added to the anaesthetic solution to enhance the spread of the anaesthetic through the orbital tissues and the speed of onset and quality of the block. This may be of use in younger patients whose denser orbital fascia may reduce spread of anaesthetic from the injection site but is not necessary in older patients with attenuated connective tissue.

Any of the local anaesthetics used can produce toxic systemic effects if used in overdose or accidentally injected intravenously. It is therefore important to know the maximum 'safe' dose of anaesthetic and to realize that this may be considerably reduced in frail elderly patients (Table 5.1).

Sedation

Although careful explanation, gentle handling during the block and a sympathetic approach will allow most patients to manage corneal procedures under local anaesthesia, some patients require sedation.

1. Oral
Oral administration of a short-acting benzodiazepine such as temazepam 10–20 mg/kg 30 minutes prior to administration of local anaesthesia and surgery provides simple sedation for young fit patients. The major drawbacks are unpredictable levels of sedation and over-sedation in the elderly causing desaturation and confusion.

2. Intravenous
Intravenous sedation with the short-acting benzodiazepine, midazolam, can be performed just prior to the anaesthetic block and carefully

titrated to maintain cooperation at all times, a usual total dose being 1–3 mg. It can be used successfully in elderly patients in very small doses, given very slowly, total dose being 0.5–1.0 mg. The anaesthetic agent propofol can also be used in sub-anaesthetic doses, but care must be taken not to lose the airway.

Day-case anaesthesia

Patient selection
The criteria used to decide which patients are suitable for day-case surgery may be divided into surgical, medical and social.

Surgical criteria

1. *Length of operation.* Although initial recommendations were to limit day-case operations to 30–40 minutes, the use of newer anaesthetic agents allows rapid recovery from general anaesthesia even after procedures lasting up to 2 hours. Obviously, the limiting factor with local anaesthesia is the time for which the block itself will work and patient tolerance.
2. *Site of operation.* Corneal surgery causes little systemic upset for the patient and comes under the same category as body surface surgery as regards suitability for day-case surgery.
3. *Postoperative pain* must be controllable with simple oral analgesics. This is the case with most corneal procedures. Padding of the eye contributes to postoperative comfort.
4. *Postoperative complications* need to be few if the patient is to go home on the same day. The patient must be able to cope with the postoperative care of the eye. If serious complications are anticipated or the eye requires intensive treatment postoperatively, then the patient is best treated on an inpatient basis.

Medical criteria
Day-case patients must be as carefully assessed preoperatively as those for inpatient treatment. A written tick sheet to assess past medical history, drug therapy and current health could be filled in at the booking clinic by medical or nursing staff. Preoperative investigations, such as urinalysis, blood pressure measurement and blood tests could be performed at this time. Only patients that fall into Class 1 and 2 of the classification of physical status adopted by the American Society of Anesthesiologists (see Appendix 5.1) are suitable for day-care

treatment. Physician referral may allow control of a medical condition so that a patient moves up into Class 2 and can be treated on a day-care basis.

Social criteria

1. *Distance* from hospital should only be about 10–12 miles to reduce patient travelling time to less than 1 hour. Hostel care providing for an overnight stay on the preoperative night and/or postoperative night might solve this problem for a hospital in a large city.

2. *Transport*. The patient should preferably be transported by private car. This obviously depends on availability of parking near the hospital.

3. *Escort*. The patient must be escorted home by a responsible adult. This should also hold for all but the most minor procedures under local anaesthesia.

4. *General practitioner*. The patient must be registered with a general practitioner at the address to which he will be returning. The general practitioner must be informed by letter that the patient is to be admitted on a day-care basis, as he will be discharged into his care.

5. *Home care* must be adequate to allow proper postoperative care of the patient.

A tick sheet to be filled in by medical or nursing staff is the best way to ensure that only patients who fulfil these criteria are admitted for day-case surgery.

Preoperative instructions

The patient must be given clear instructions both verbally and written. These should include: the need for 6 hours' starvation prior to general anaesthesia; which medication should be continued on the morning of surgery; and details of where and when they should arrive. A visit to the day-care ward after booking will allay many patient fears.

Day of surgery

The patient should be assessed by the surgeon and anaesthetist who will perform the procedure. It is recommended in the Royal College of Surgeon's report on day-care surgery that both the surgeon and anaesthetist are senior members of staff. The patient should be cared for on a dedicated day ward, with staff especially trained to deal with day-care patients. The ward should be situated close to the operating theatres to allow easy access for the surgeon and anaesthetist.

Anaesthesia

Anaesthesia may be local or general as appropriate. No premedication is given as a routine. For general anaesthesia, shorter acting agents are used and care taken to minimize postoperative pain, nausea and vomiting.

Postoperative recovery and discharge

A clear set of discharge criteria should be established for the day-care unit and documented for each patient:

1. The patient must be able to swallow and cough.
2. The patient's vital signs must be stable for at least 1 hour.
3. The patient must be alert and orientated in person, place and time.
4. The patient must be able to take oral fluids.
5. The patient should be able to pass urine.
6. The patient should be able to dress and walk without assistance.
7. The patient must have a responsible adult to escort him home.
8. The patient must be given verbal and written postoperative instructions and a telephone number in case of problems.

The patient should be seen and discharged by the surgeon and anaesthetist involved in his care. If necessary, arrangements must be made for admission of the patient.

APPENDIX 5.1: THE CLASSIFICATION OF PHYSICAL STATUS ADOPTED BY THE AMERICAN SOCIETY OF ANESTHESIOLOGISTS

Class 1

There is no organic, physiological, biochemical or psychiatric disturbance. The pathologic process for which the operation is to be performed is localized and is not a systemic disturbance.

Examples: a fit patient with inguinal hernia; fibroid uterus in an otherwise fit woman.

Class 2

Mild to moderate systemic disturbance caused either by the condition to be treated surgically or by other pathological processes.

Examples: patients with non- or only slightly limiting organic heart disease; mild diabetes, essential hypertension or anaemia. Some might choose to list the extremes of age here, either the neonate or the octogenarian, even though no discernible disease is present. Extreme obesity, heavy smoking and chronic bronchitis are included.

Class 3

Severe systemic disturbance or disease from whatever cause, even though it may not be possible to define the degree of disability with finality.

Examples: severely limiting organic heart disease; severe diabetes with vascular complications; moderate to severe degrees of pulmonary insufficiency; angina pectoris or healed myocardial infarction.

Class 4

Indicative of the patient with severe systemic disorder already life-threatening, not always correctable by the operative procedure.

Examples: patients with organic heart disease showing marked signs of cardiac insufficiency, the anginal syndrome or active myocarditis; advanced degrees of pulmonary, hepatic, renal or endocrine insufficiency.

Class 5

The moribund patient who has little chance of survival, but is submitted to operation in desperation.

Examples: the burst abdominal aneurysm with profound shock; major cerebral trauma with rapidly increasing intracranial pressure; massive pulmonary embolus. Most of these patients require operation as a resuscitative measure with little if any anaesthesia.

Emergency operation (E)

Any patient in one of the classes listed who is operated upon as an emergency is considered to be in poorer physical condition. The letter E is placed beside the numerical classification.

Example: the patient with a hitherto uncomplicated hernia now incarcerated and associated with nausea and vomiting is classified 1E.

6

Corneal biopsy

INDICATIONS

Corneal biopsy may be indicated for the diagnosis of Bowen's disease or for other infiltrative lesions and cases of presumed microbial keratitis where a corneal scrape has not yielded a positive result. In the former cases, the biopsy need only be deep enough to include a portion of the abnormal feature, but, in a case of presumed infection (Fig. 6.1), the biopsy needs to be as deep as it can be, to cover the possibility that acanthamoeba is the infective agent. The active acanthamoebae burrow deeply into the cornea, feeding on the nuclei of keratocytes and leaving dead keratocytes in their trail. This excites an inflammatory response. Thus, if only the abscess is biopsied, the organism may not be found (Fig. 6.2).

TECHNIQUE

Epithelial biopsy

For corneal intra-epithelial neoplasia and other lesions such as malignant melanoma, which may not yet have invaded Bowman's membrane, the biopsy should remain confined solely to the epithelium. The area to be biopsied should be marked *very lightly* with a trephine of appropriate size or with a blade which is not too sharp. A dulled razor fragment is ideal for this, if a freehand dissection is necessary. The edge of the

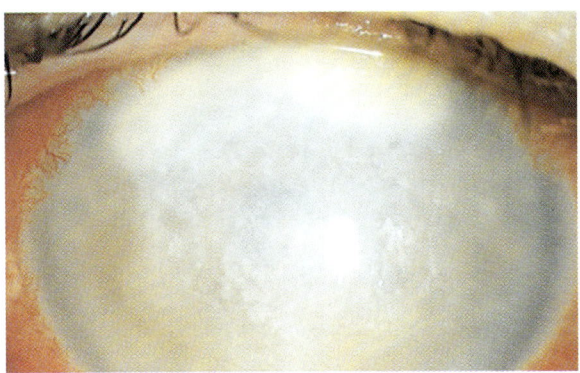

Fig. 6.1.

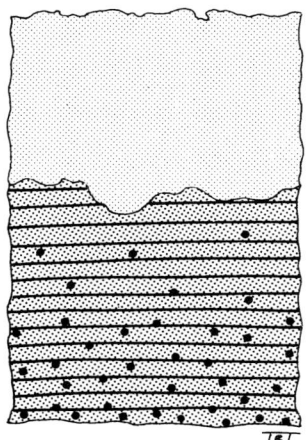

Fig. 6.2.

epithelium is gently rolled back using a dry cellulose sponge and a Paufique knife can be used to extend the dissection. Very often the epithelial lesion will lack structure and tend to fragment but that will not affect the ability to examine them histologically. It is helpful not to place the tiny specimens in a large pot of preservative.

In Bowen's disease, a superficial keratectomy including all the clinically involved epithelium may be performed; if limbal or conjunctival tissue is involved, this may also be included. In this condition, there is no need to cut beneath Bowman's membrane, since the carcinoma is not invasive.

Deep corneal biopsy

The technique of deep corneal biopsy is essentially the same in all cases, but since it is slightly more complex to biopsy an ulcer, this will be described.

1. All antibiotics and other treatment should be discontinued for 24–48 hours, to increase the chances of culturing an organism.

2. The superficial slough should be debrided. This can be plated out on to blood agar. A scrape may be taken from the surface of the ulcer for direct microscopy.

3. If possible, the biopsy should avoid the area of visual axis and the edge of the abscess should be included in the specimen (Fig. 6.3). A disposable 2-, 3- or 4-mm trephine punch is ideal for marking the tissue, and the cut is deepened with a blade.

4. A lamellar dissection is then completed with a Paufique knife (Fig. 6.4).

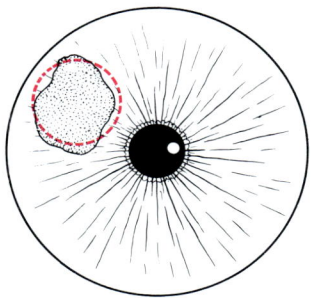

Fig. 6.3.

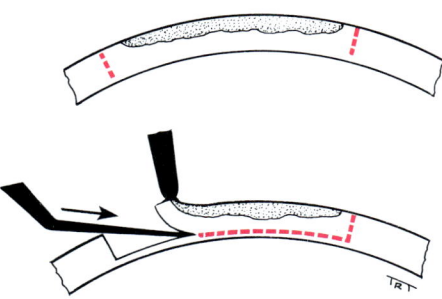

Fig. 6.4.

It is always wise to be prepared for perforation when dealing with necrotic tissue, and donor material should be at hand in case conversion to a penetrating keratoplasty is necessary. For this reason, it is preferable for a deep corneal biopsy to be performed under general anaesthesia. This has the further advantage that no topical drops need be used, thereby increasing the chances of obtaining a positive culture. Should local anaesthesia be chosen, it is important that all solutions used are free of preservative.

Following excision, the specimen should immediately be sent to the laboratory, where it can be processed without delay. Infected tissue will be divided in two, one part for histology and the other for maceration and plating out for culture.

Conjunctival biopsy

There are many reasons why the conjunctiva may be biopsied. Usually this involves removing a small piece for diagnostic purposes but occasionally a small lesion may be removed in toto in an excision biopsy. The siting of the biopsy may be of importance. Follicles in the tarsal conjunctiva may be the only abnormality and they must therefore be chosen but, in general, the depth of the fornix should be avoided since symblepharon may form subsequently. If the diagnosis appears to be cicatricial conjunctivitis then a site on the bulbar conjunctiva 3–4 mm behind the limbus in the lower temporal quadrant is safest.

After applying proxymetacaine to the conjunctival sac, a small bleb is raised with 0.5% warmed plain lignocaine through a 27 gauge needle. The conjunctiva is grasped with a pair of notched forceps and a small piece of conjunctiva approximately 2 mm in diameter is cut off with scissors. Suturing is not necessary.

If a large excision biopsy has been deemed necessary, the bare area may be covered with a free conjunctival graft from the fellow eye (see Ch. 17).

Section B
Penetrating keratoplasty

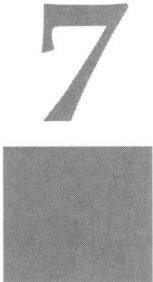

Donor preparation for penetrating keratoplasty

Donor material may be made available to the surgeon from his Eye Bank either as a whole donor eye stored in a moist chamber at 4°C, or as a corneo-scleral disc which has been prepared from a whole donor eye by the Eye Bank and stored in a preservative medium. The technique for the surgeon will be different in each case.

Preparation from a whole donor eye

1. The eye is removed from its container and immersed in a solution of 0.5% Soframycin or some equivalent antibiotic solution for 3 minutes. The eye is then gently removed from the solution and is thoroughly rinsed with isotonic saline.

2. The eye is now placed in the donor eye stand (Fig. 7.1). The stand favoured by the authors is one designed by Pierse and Steele and has the advantage of simple adjustment of the intraocular pressure. The eye is secured in the stand with the corneal surface uppermost, and the tension of the eye adjusted to approximate to normal.

3. Using a cellulose swab, loose epithelium is removed from the surface of the cornea. It is undesirable to scrape at the epithelium with the blade of a knife or use any degree of force for this removal process. Epithelium which is adherent to its underlying basement membrane is best left in place.

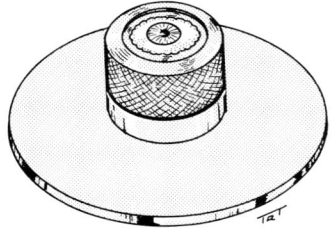

Fig. 7.1.

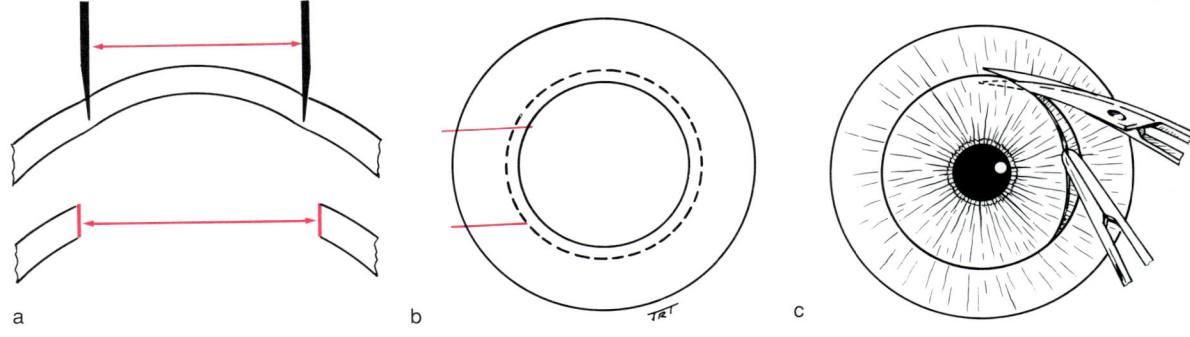

a   b   c

Fig. 7.2.

4. Selecting a hollow trephine of the appropriate dimension, the edge is carefully examined under the microscope to ensure that it is both clean and evenly sharp. The cornea is trephined to approximately three-quarters or four-fifths of corneal thickness under microscopic control and with the trephine centred on the cornea (Fig. 7.2a).

5. The trephine is now removed and the precise diameter of the trephined disc measured with a pair of callipers (Fig. 7.2b). It is quite possible to produce markedly different sized buttons with the same trephine but differing external and intraocular pressure and differing corneal rigidity.

6. The corneal disc is now removed from the surrounding cornea using a diamond knife or curved corneal scissors. Care must be taken at this stage to *avoid undercutting* the corneal graft wound. It is also important to *avoid any bending* of the donor disc, as this is damaging to the corneal endothelium. Care must also be taken to ensure that the *edge of the corneal disc is vertical* (Fig. 7.2c).

When removed, the disc should be left in the donor eye supported on a bed of visco-elastic fluid until it is ready for transfer to the recipient.

Preparation from a stored disc

1. The corneo-scleral disc is carefully removed from its container and placed with its endothelial surface uppermost on a shaped silicone-rubber cutting block (Fig. 7.3).

2. Using an ultrasharp disposable trephine blade of size of 0.25 mm larger than is required for the patient's graft bed, the trephine is gently applied to the endothelial surface of the corneal disc. Firm,

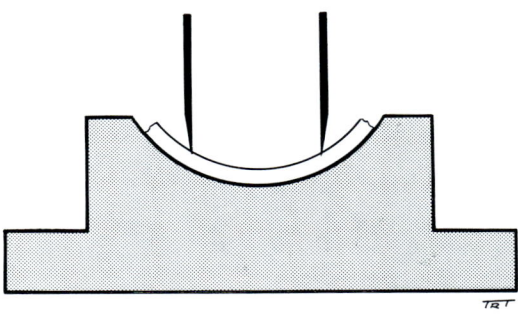

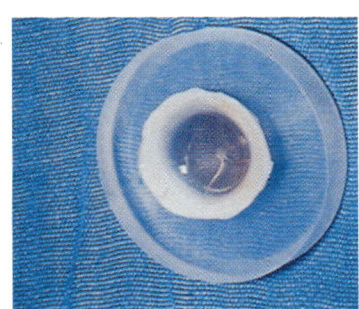

Fig. 7.3.   Fig. 7.4.

even pressure is applied to drive the trephine through the disc in a single smooth movement (Fig. 7.4).

3. The trephine is removed and this will usually leave the cut disc on the cutting block. The corneo-scleral rim is usually left adherent to the outer surface of the disposable trephine. The surface of the cut disc is now kept moist using either visco-elastic fluid or a few drops of the storage medium.

The disc should now be left on the cutting block under a cover until it is required for transfer to the recipient.

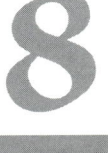

8

Routine penetrating keratoplasty

An hour or so before transfer to theatre, the patient's eye for grafting will have three or four drops of 4% pilocarpine instilled to produce an intense miosis. Following skin preparation, the eye for surgery is draped using an adhesive plastic drape which is divided across the eye midway between the open lid margins. The flaps of drape material so formed are then tucked under the lid margin using a wire speculum to preclude the lid margins and eyelashes from the surgical field (Fig. 8.1).

SURGICAL TECHNIQUE

1. Sutures are inserted through the insertions of the superior and inferior recti. These sutures are then clipped with artery forceps to the surgical drape to maintain the eye in a vertical position with respect to the surgical microscope (Fig. 8.2).

2. A scleral supporting ring, preferably a broad titanium ring, should be sutured to the sclera and as close to the limbus as is convenient. This step is not essential for all patients, but is particularly helpful when operating on eyes which are already aphakic or which may become aphakic or pseudophakic in the course of the surgical

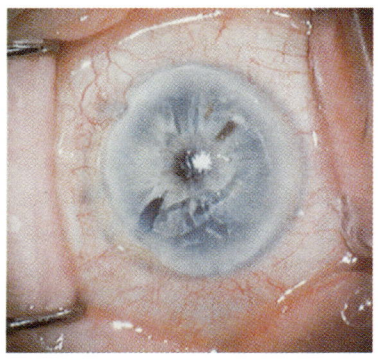

Fig. 8.1.

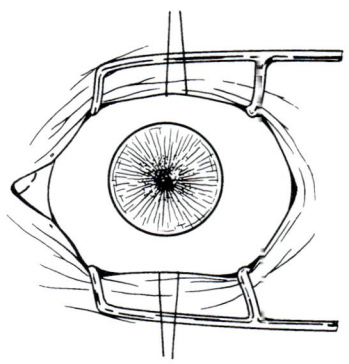

Fig. 8.2.

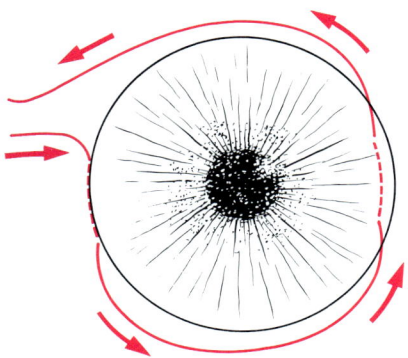

Fig. 8.3.

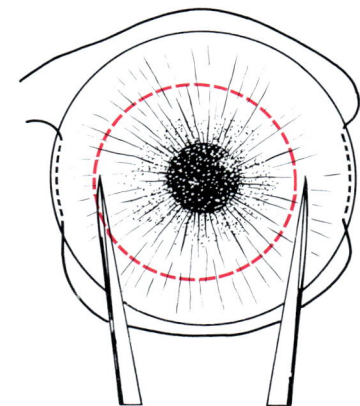

Fig. 8.4.

procedure. The ring supports the anterior segment of the eye during surgery so as to limit scleral collapse and distortion of the graft wound opening.

3. Using 7/0 silk, one or two overlay sutures are inserted. These are so placed at the limbus that when they are tied at a later stage they will support the centre of the graft securely (Fig. 8.3).

4. The overlay sutures are loosened and arranged around the limbus so as to leave the cornea clearly exposed.

5. Using a pair of callipers, the surgeon determines the size of the graft required (Fig. 8.4). It should be noted that very small grafts may give rise to high degrees of postoperative astigmatism, whereas large grafts, necessarily closer to the limbal vasculature, are at greater risk of subsequent rejection. Most grafts are between 7 and 8 mm in diameter.

6. Preparation of the donor disc. See Chapter 7.

7. *Removal of the host disc.* Using a hollow trephine of the size required, the blade is placed upon the corneal surface, without rotation but with gentle pressure, so as to make a mark on the epithelial surface. On removal of the trephine, one can then see whether the graft will be properly placed. The mark should also be measured to ensure that the size of the graft is correct for the size of the donor disc already obtained. Once the positioning has been corrected (if necessary), the trephine is used to cut the stroma to approximately half depth. The trephine is once more removed and the size of the trephination re-measured. *It is most important to ensure that the size of the trephined disc is not larger than the size of the donor disc already cut.*

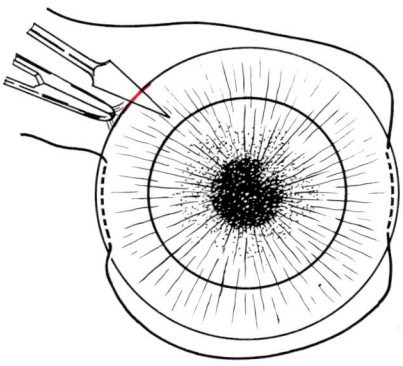

Fig. 8.5.

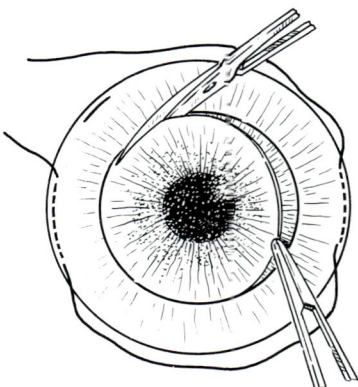

Fig. 8.6.

Should such a discrepancy occur, a smaller trephine must be selected at this stage for the host eye.

8. A paracentesis is performed, wide enough to admit a fine cannula to the anterior chamber. This opening is usually most conveniently situated in the lower temporal quadrant, where access is easy (Fig. 8.5).

9. Using a diamond knife and scissors, the host disc is now removed completely (Fig. 8.6).

10. The anterior surface of the lens and iris are covered with a layer of visco-elastic fluid.

11. With great care and being sure not to touch the endothelial surface, the donor disc is transferred from its holder and gently placed on the recipient's eye. The overlay suture, or sutures, are tied to secure the disc in position (Fig. 8.7). If the donor disc has any peripheral opacity due to arcus in the donor, this area should be placed in the uppermost part of the circumference where it will be occluded by the eyelid postoperatively.

12. Using 10/0 nylon suture material and sharp, 6 mm cutting edge needles, four interrupted sutures are placed across the graft wound at the 12, 3, 6 and 9 o'clock positions (Fig. 8.7). These sutures need only be short and superficial, as they will be removed before the end of the operation. They will, however, secure the cornea in its correct position. Great care must be taken when placing the second of these interrupted sutures, which the surgeon will use to distribute and fix the disc within the host bed. Errors at this stage are likely to have long-lasting effects upon corneal shape.

13. The overlay sutures are removed.

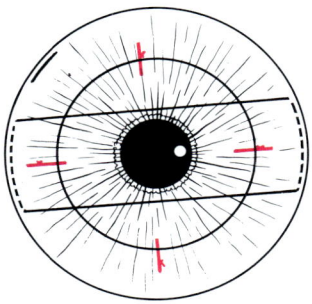

Fig. 8.7.

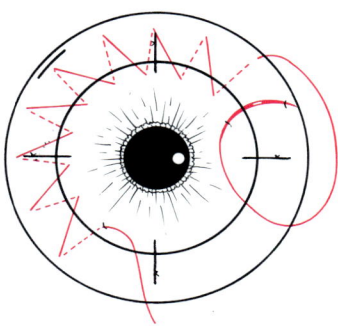

Fig. 8.8.

14. The donor disc should be supported on a thin layer of visco-elastic fluid. If necessary, the depth of this layer may now be increased by injecting further visco-elastic fluid through the paracentesis. It is neither necessary nor desirable to have the anterior chamber completely filled with visco-elastic fluid.

15. The definitive sutures are now placed. The graft may be secured using either continuous or interrupted sutures:

   a. *Continuous.* A continuous suture is conveniently started in the upper temporal quadrant. The first bite of the suture is from the depth of the wound into host stroma only. Subsequent bites then include both the donor disc and the host tissue (Fig. 8.8) until the last bite, placed exactly opposite the first, which will be through donor disc only, and emerging from the wound. Suture bites may either be placed radially to the graft wound, or be introduced torque-free. Suture bites should be short and deep into the donor disc, but longer and deep into the host tissue. The length of the bite should be almost three times as long into the host as into the donor. Graft sutures should be at as great a depth as the surgeon can conveniently achieve. They should not, however, be through and through, as this gives rise to leakage of aqueous along the suture track.

   After the continuous suture has been completed, the suture ends will emerge together through the wound. A simple two-loop tie is made so that the knot will sink into the depth of the wound. The four temporary interrupted sutures are now removed, and the continuous suture is tightened around its circumference to achieve a leak-free wound. Before completing the knot, the anterior chamber is deepened with normal saline or balanced salt solution. This reveals any area of leakage requiring further suture tightening. At this stage, obvious

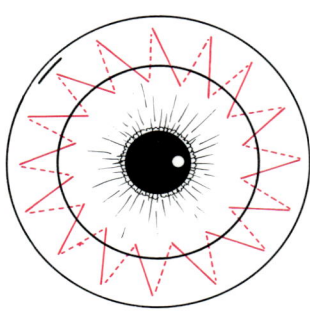 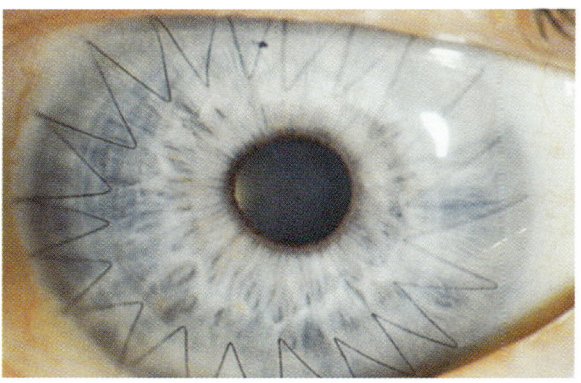

Fig. 8.9.

defects of curvature will be visible or demonstrable, and are corrected by adjustments to the suture tension.

A simple ring device or Maloney keratoscope held over the moistened corneal surface can be used as a surgical keratometer to demonstrate the presence of astigmatic errors, and is surprisingly accurate.

When even curvatures and a leak-free wound have been achieved, the knot is completed and the suture ends cut close to the knot (Fig. 8.9).

b. *Interrupted sutures*. Some surgeons use these for preference in all cases. They should, however, always be used for children, for emergency corneal grafting when the eye is inflamed, and in patients where there is considerable vascularization of the host corneal tissue. Under these circumstances, the host stroma is inclined to be soft and less able to withstand suture tensions throughout the usual period of healing. Individual sutures which loosen can easily be removed, but the premature loosening of a segment of continuous suture can be inconvenient. There are usually 16 interrupted sutures, evenly distributed around the circumference of the corneal graft. Smaller grafts may be secured with fewer sutures and larger grafts with more (Fig. 8.10).

c. *Mixed continuous and interrupted sutures*. Some surgeons believe that a combination of interrupted and continuous sutures has the advantage of control over astigmatism during the period of graft healing (Fig. 8.11).

At the conclusion of the insertion of all interrupted sutures, the anterior chamber is deepened with normal saline or

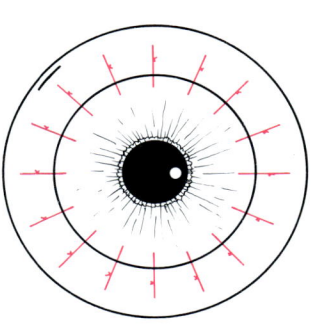
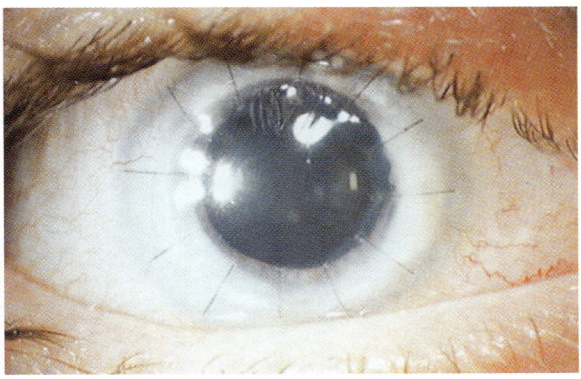

Fig. 8.10.

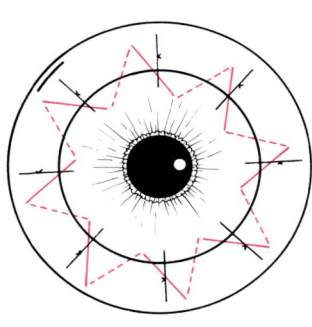
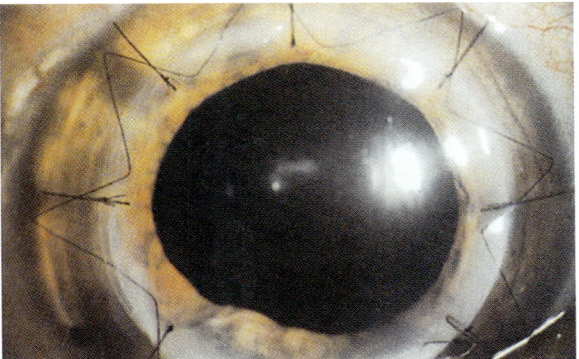

Fig. 8.11.

balanced salt solution and the wound checked for accuracy of closure and even tensions. Again, the simple keratometric device is useful to show that individual sutures are not producing distortion. Interrupted sutures should be cut close to the knot and all knots then turned into the suture track.

d. *Double running suture* (Figs 8.12–8.16). Some surgeons recommend the double running suture as the technique of choice in uncomplicated cases, arguing that it produces less astigmatism. This is not necessarily so in our experience but it may produce less astigmatism while the sutures are in place. The technique is somewhat more difficult at first and appears awkward since the suture is crossing the wound at a very oblique angle.

The overlay sutures are applied as above. After the first four are inserted the overlay suture is removed. To begin with we recommend at least four pre-placed radial sutures or even eight

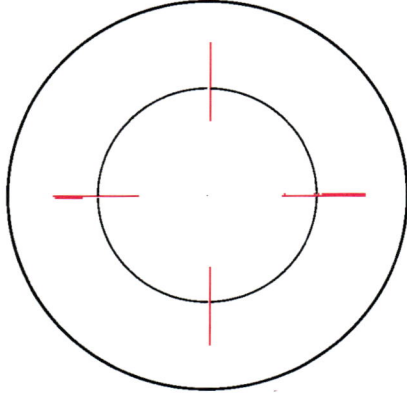

Fig. 8.12.

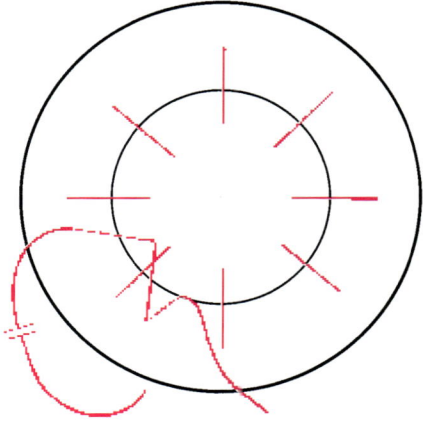

Fig. 8.13.

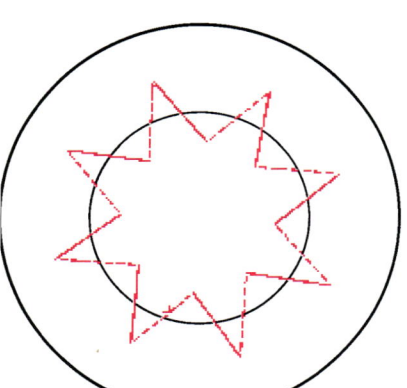

Fig. 8.14.

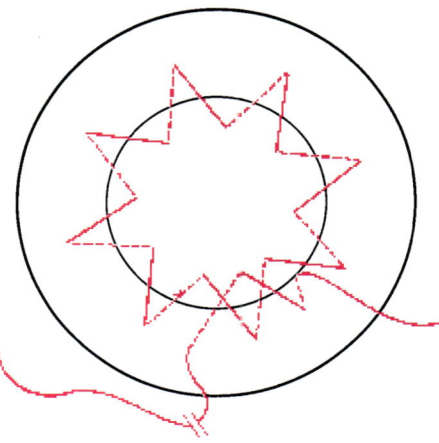

Fig. 8.15.

if in any doubt about the spacing. The first continuous suture is begun in the same way as the combined running and interrupted suture above.

When the first running suture is complete, a triple throw is passed over the short end and the tension is increased until the suture is just snug. The interrupted sutures are removed. The second suture is begun in the upper right-hand quadrant (assuming the first was begun in the upper left-hand quadrant).

This time the spacing is easier. The suture is 180° out of phase with the first one, i.e. the inner points of the second are placed opposite the outer points of the first and so on. It will be

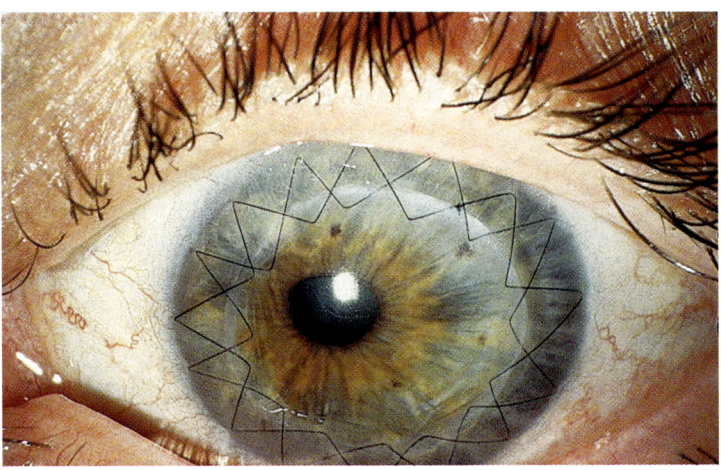

Fig. 8.16.

noted that unlike the combination interrupted and running, in this approach at no point do the sutures come into contact with one another.

Once completed a triple throw is placed on the second. The first is tightened from the knot clockwise and the knot tightened. The second is tightened from the knot anticlockwise and the knot tightened. The combination of the pattern and the careful anti-torque tightening does appear to reduce the torque on the graft. Once the wound is watertight, the astigmatism may be checked with the keratoscope and the tension adjusted accordingly. It is usual that the first suture is tighter than the second. It may be preferentially removed earlier than the second to reduce astigmatism further.

16. The scleral supporting ring and rectus sutures are removed.

17. Subconjunctival injections of steroid and antibiotic preparation are administered. The authors currently use betamethasone sodium 4 mg and cefuroxime 125 mg or gentamicin 10 mg.

18. The eye is dressed with a Melolin pad and a Cartella shield, if the lid will not close passively, or as a matter of personal preference an eye pad until the morning of the following day when the dressing is removed.

PERIOPERATIVE COMPLICATIONS

Haemorrhage

Bleeding may occur from cut corneal vessels. Persistent bleeding is a nuisance because it gives rise to clots in the anterior chamber which can then lead to the formation of adhesions between the anterior iris surface and the back of the graft wound. Bleeding may be inhibited by the instillation of adrenaline eye drops 1/1000 or 1/10 000 before the anterior chamber is opened. If bleeding persists after the anterior chamber is opened, it can usually be stopped by the application of visco-elastic fluid to the bleeding vessel. *Under no circumstances should the surgeon be tempted to cauterise bleeding vessels at the wound edge.*

As with any intraocular procedure, the surgeon may occasionally be faced with the potential disaster of an expulsive choroidal haemorrhage. During corneal grafting this will be easily detected by the forward protrusion of the ocular contents through the graft wound. If it is suspected, the site of the haemorrhage should be sought by inspection of the fundus through the surgical microscope, and a sclerotomy in the appropriate area performed without delay. Sclerotomy on its own will not be sufficient unless the corneal wound can be closed efficiently and quickly.

Damage to the lens

In the event of damage to the anterior lens surface during removal of the diseased host disc, the surgeon must proceed to extracapsular cataract extraction and probably the insertion of a posterior chamber intraocular lens.

Wound leakage

If, after completing the suturing process and the tying of the knot, it is discovered that the wound is continuing to leak, further supplementary interrupted 10/0 sutures are required. Where a continuous suture has already been inserted, great care must be taken not to damage it with the cutting edge of the needle.

Synechiae

Where corneal disease has been associated with the development of adhesions between the iris and the posterior corneal surface, these must be gently separated or dissected free with the minimum of damage to the iris. Wherever possible, care should be taken to avoid the excision of iris tissue.

POSTOPERATIVE MANAGEMENT

Most grafts are treated with steroid and antibiotic drops only. Mydriatic agents are not usually required, unless the patient can be expected to have a significant degree of postoperative anterior uveitis. Drops are continued on a gradually diminishing scale for 6–12 months postoperatively, depending upon the patient's progress. Regular monitoring is required for the early detection of complications. A spectacle or contact lens correction may be prescribed when necessary 3 months postoperatively.

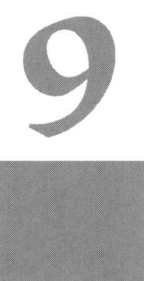

The penetrating rotational autograft

INDICATIONS

Occasionally, a patient's vision will be limited by the presence of a central scar across the visual axis. If the extent of this scar is limited, e.g. linear, and leaves a wide area of healthy unscarred corneal tissue in the periphery, the patient may well be suitable for a rotational autograft procedure. The principle of such a technique is to identify a circle which includes both healthy periphery and the central scarring. By mobilizing the circle, one can rotate the scar to the periphery and the clear healthy tissue to the visual axis.

PREOPERATIVE PLANNING

When a rotational autograft is being contemplated, it is wise to map out the features of the cornea on paper to scale, and then by trial and error to define the best size and position for the autograft. The graft size is often extremely critical. The graft edge must be sufficiently far from the visual axis to minimize postoperative glare. Too large a graft may not, however, allow the scar to be rotated away.

SURGICAL TECHNIQUE

The early stages of patient preparation and surgical technique are the same as for a routine penetrating keratoplasty up to the time of the insertion of the rectus sutures. Further steps in the procedure are as follows:

1. *Confirmation of graft site and size.* The nature of the technique means that it is seldom possible to perform a rotational autograft greater than 7 mm in diameter; most satisfactory autografts are of 6–6.5 mm diameter only. Grafts smaller than this are likely to be affected by severe astigmatic error and are not advised. Using the trephine of the chosen size, a mark is made on the corneal epithelium where it is proposed to perform the rotational autograft (Fig. 9.1). The

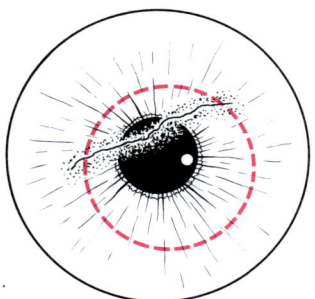

Fig. 9.1.

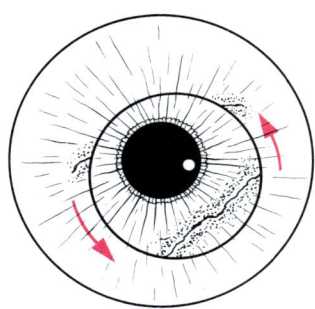

Fig. 9.2.

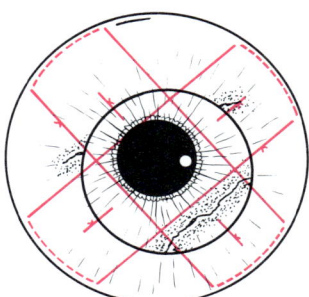

Fig. 9.3.

preoperative planning is thus confirmed on the table and any last adjustments made. A firm indentation in the corneal epithelium is then made, delineating the intended graft.

2. *Overlay sutures*. As the autograft will be eccentric, the overlay sutures need to be positioned so as to give the graft the necessary support.

3. *Trephination*. Using the chosen trephine, the corneal mark is now deepened to approximately half corneal depth.

4. A paracentesis is made at a convenient point at the limbus.

5. The corneal disc is mobilized using fine tissue-holding forceps and a diamond knife. Great care must be taken during this process to ensure that the corneal wound remains normal to the surface round the entire circumference. Corneal curved scissors are best avoided, as they may well damage the endothelial surface on one or other side of the wound. While using the diamond knife to mobilize the cornea, care must be taken to avoid damaging the underlying iris or lens epithelium. Visco-elastic fluid should be used to separate these surfaces.

6. Once the wound is completed, the disc is grasped with two pairs of fine toothed forceps on each side and is then gently lifted and rotated into its new position (Fig. 9.2). Care should be taken to ensure that the disc is not bent and that the endothelium does not come into contact with other tissues during the rotation process.

7. Keeping a layer of visco-elastic material between the corneal endothelium and the iris, the overlay sutures are gently tied to support the graft in its new position (Fig. 9.3).

8. Four short superficial interrupted sutures are inserted as stay sutures.

9. The graft is secured in position using either 12 or 16 interrupted nylon sutures (Fig. 9.4) or a continuous suture. This requires a careful and atraumatic technique to avoid corneal bending and endothelial touch. The surgeon must remember that the patient's endothelium is

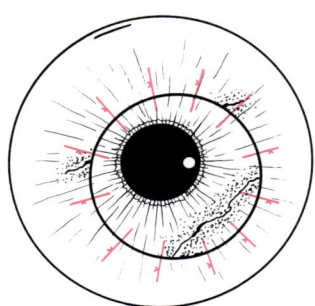

Fig. 9.4.

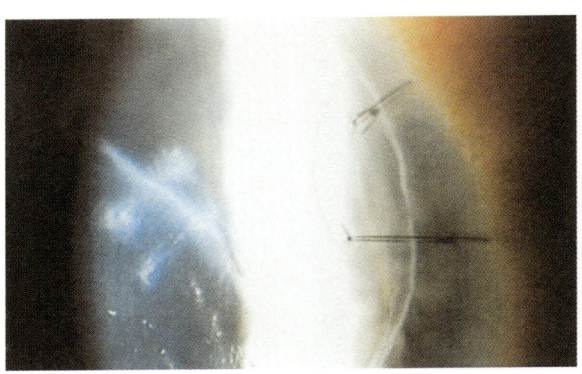

Fig. 9.5.

already compromised by the preceding pathology and that it will readily decompensate if mishandled.

The remainder of the surgical process is as for the routine penetrating keratoplasty (Fig. 9.5). As these patients are not at risk of an immune rejection, it is usually not necessary to maintain the steroid dosage for more than about 6 weeks postoperatively. This will ensure more rapid healing of the corneal wound, and will permit earlier removal of the graft suture without the same risk of misadventure due to inadequate healing.

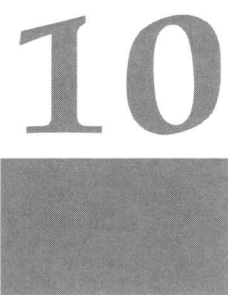

Combined penetrating keratoplasty and lens surgery

INDICATION

Where the need for corneal grafting co-exists with the presence of a significant amount of cataract, the two problems are best dealt with simultaneously by combined surgery. Because of the advantages for the stability of the anterior segment, the posterior lens capsule should be preserved and, wherever possible, used for the support of a posterior chamber intraocular lens. Intracapsular cataract extraction carries the disadvantage of vitreous gaining access to the anterior chamber, where it can pose a hazard for the corneal graft and the control of intraocular pressure. As usual, vitreous displacement can also be associated with the development of retinal complications.

For these reasons, the procedure described below is for *penetrating keratoplasty with extracapsular cataract extraction and placement of a posterior chamber intraocular lens.*

PREOPERATIVE MEDICATION

Unlike the case for other patients undergoing corneal grafting or cataract surgery, the usual preoperative drops are not helpful. A wide preoperative mydriasis can make the corneal graft difficult, whereas an intense miosis will prejudice the safe management of the cataract. At the time of the induction of anaesthesia, one or two drops only of cyclopentolate 1% without preservative may be instilled into the eye.

SURGICAL TECHNIQUE

1. The eye is prepared as for routine penetrating keratoplasty, and superior and inferior rectus sutures are inserted.
2. An anterior scleral supporting ring is sutured into place (Fig. 10.1).
3. The procedure is as for a normal penetrating keratoplasty up to the time of the removal of the diseased host disc, then using a pair of fine scissors, a circle of anterior capsule is excised of approximately 6 mm

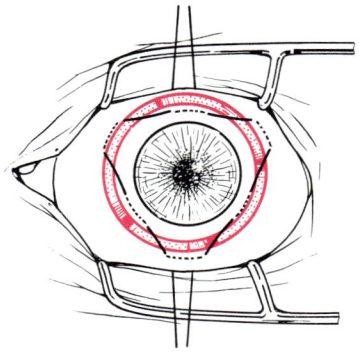

Fig. 10.1.

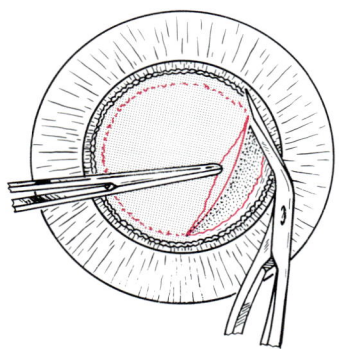

Fig. 10.2.

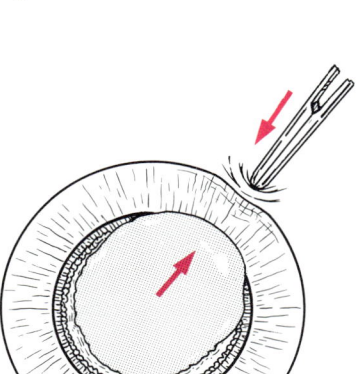

Fig. 10.3.

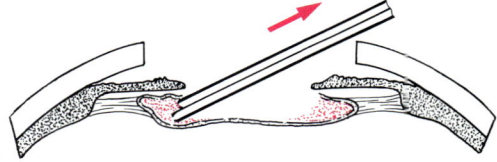

Fig. 10.4.

diameter (Fig. 10.2). By gentle pressure (within the ring) on the anterior sclera, the lens nucleus will easily be expressed and removed (Fig. 10.3). Using either a co-axial or a Simco aspiration/irrigation cannula, the remaining cortex of the lens is gently teased from the periphery of the capsular bag (Fig. 10.4). This process requires great care. It is extremely easy to damage the posterior capsule, and time should be taken for the process. Remaining cortex may easily be demonstrated by gently sweeping the edge of the iris from side to side to reveal peripheral lens matter against the red reflex. The authors advise excising the anterior capsule with scissors rather than by capsulorhexis as preferred with phacoemulsification. These patients are often elderly with large hard nuclei. Attempts to express such a nucleus through a capsular opening can easily lead to zonular rupture and extrusion of the whole lens.

4. When the cortex is completely removed, an intraocular lens is placed

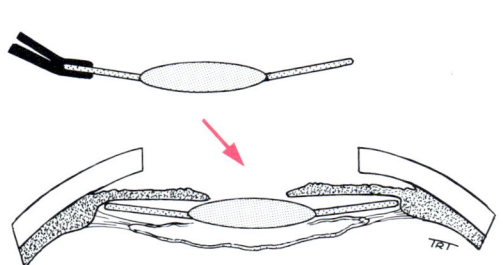

Fig. 10.5.

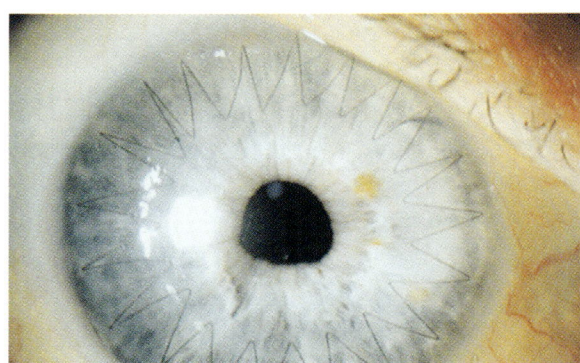

Fig. 10.6.

into the posterior chamber, making no effort to achieve bag placement. The lens will be supported by the ciliary sulcus. Attempts to achieve bag placement in this situation are too easily followed postoperatively by one haptic escaping and leading to lens decentration. The lens should be carefully centred so that the optical centre coincides with the pupillary opening (Fig. 10.5).

5. The iris should now be gently irrigated with Miochol to achieve as tight a miosis as possible.

6. The anterior surface of the iris and the intraocular implant are covered with viscoelastic fluid, and the process of corneal grafting is resumed as before. Figure 10.6 shows the postoperative appearance.

Penetrating keratoplasty for aphakia

For the aphakic eye, the technique described for penetrating keratoplasty requires some modification:

1. An anterior scleral support ring should always be applied after the insertion of the superior and inferior rectus sutures. The aphakic eye is liable to scleral collapse, which can alter the stability of the anterior segment and lead to serious distortion of the corneal graft wound. This, in turn, leads to less atraumatic techniques than are desirable to secure wound closure. The anterior scleral supporting ring limits this risk.

2. Where the previous lens surgery has been by an intracapsular method, it is usual to find vitreous in the anterior chamber. The corneal disc may be attached to this vitreous, and needs to be cut free gently with vitreous scissors. Using a mechanical vitrector, an open sky vitrectomy should be continued until the posterior iris surface and pupillary opening are free of contact with the remaining vitreous (Fig. 11.1). Care should be taken to avoid unduly high suction pressures during this procedure, to avoid retinal traction.

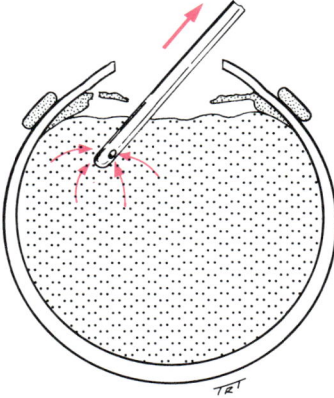

Fig. 11.1.

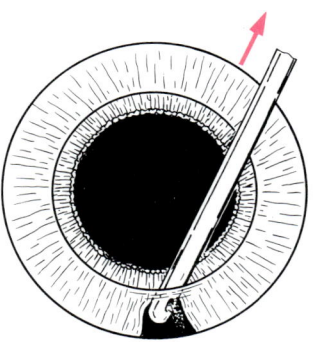

Fig. 11.2.

Once sufficient vitreous has been removed, the space may be filled using visco-elastic material or balanced saline solution without risk of vitreous re-entering the anterior chamber. Where previous iridectomies have been performed, it is essential to ensure that vitreous is not transversing the opening. The mechanical vitrector should be passed through the iridectomy, and vitrectomy continued until the edges of the iridectomy are free of vitreous contact (Fig. 11.2).

3. *Insertion of the intraocular lens.* The surgeon may decide that the opportunity should be taken during penetrating keratoplasty to correct the patient's aphakic state by inserting an appropriate intraocular lens. The techniques for these procedures are dealt with in the section on penetrating keratoplasty for pseudophakia (Ch. 12).

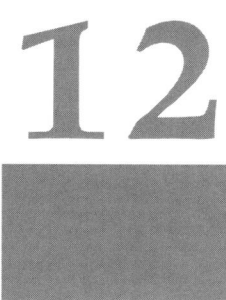

12

Penetrating keratoplasty for pseudophakia

INDICATION

When grafting is required for eyes already pseudophakic, the invariable indication is endothelial decompensation. In most cases this will be iatrogenic. Before proceeding with penetrating keratoplasty, the surgeon needs to determine his attitude to the intraocular implant already in place. In many cases, the style of the implant and its position in the eye may well have led to direct corneal endothelial damage and ensuing decompensation. Failure to identify these cases, and to remove or exchange the offending implants, will almost certainly lead to subsequent failure of the graft. The factors to consider are:

1. the type of previous cataract surgery, either intra- or extracapsular
2. the presence or absence of a strong posterior capsular framework
3. the type of intraocular implant already in place and its fixation
4. any history of raised intraocular pressure or frank glaucoma, whether or not it requires treatment now.

Intraocular lens removal or retention

Well-centred and stable posterior chamber intraocular lenses are best left alone. They are seldom a cause for corneal damage. Iris-fixated lenses, on the other hand, are almost certainly best removed in the opinion of these authors. For anterior chamber intraocular lenses where patients have a history of glaucoma, where the lens is demonstrably mobile, or where the patient has complained of persistent anterior segment pain since the cataract operation, the anterior chamber lens should be removed. Secure intraocular lenses, however, in the absence of these other features, are probably best left in situ, as their removal can be traumatic as well as unnecessary (Fig. 12 1).

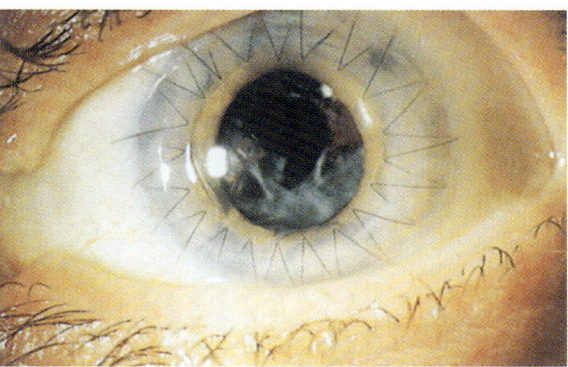

Fig. 12.1.

Intraocular lens replacement

The easiest lens to introduce under these circumstances is a posterior chamber lens, and this should always be employed where there is a strong framework of posterior capsule, even if it has previously been perforated centrally by a capsulotomy (Fig. 12.2). A preceding anterior vitrectomy may be required. It is also necessary to clear synechiae between the posterior iris surface and the capsule. This requires very gentle teasing dissection, using a combination of visco-elastic fluid and a fine, smooth-edged iris repositor. Very dense synechiae may require division with fine-bladed scissors. Where there are extensive synechiae, this process is probably best avoided and some other form of intraocular lens fixation adopted.

An anterior chamber intraocular lens of an open-loop, semi-flexible variety (Fig. 12.3) may be inserted into the angle of the anterior

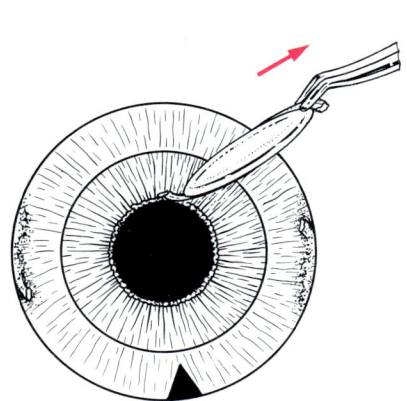

Fig. 12.2.

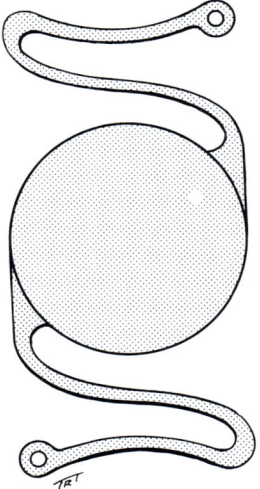

Fig. 12.3.

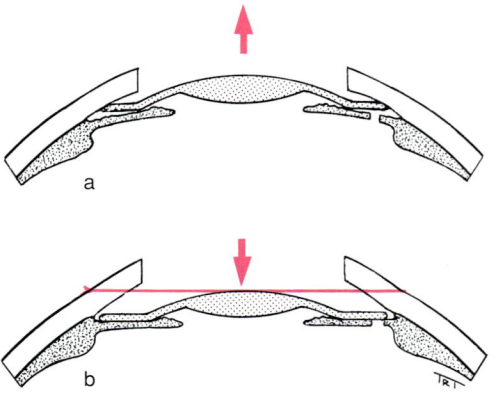

Fig. 12.4.

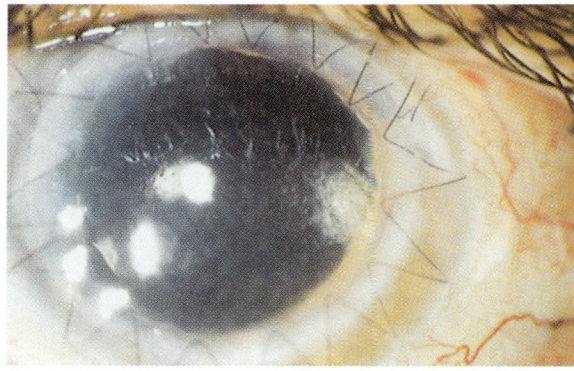

Fig. 12.5.

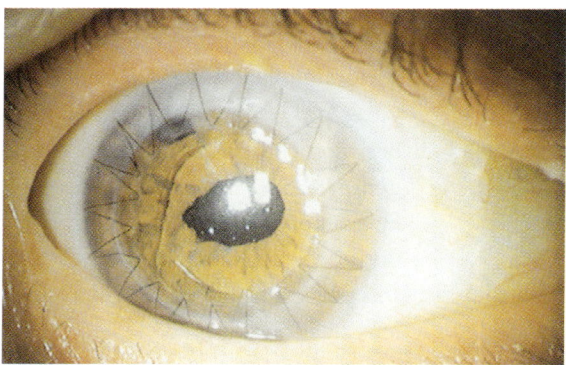

Fig. 12.6.

chamber, providing the angle is normal and there is no past history of raised intraocular pressure or glaucoma. After its insertion, and during the ensuing suturing of the corneal graft, particular care must be taken to ensure that there is no contact between the graft endothelium and the anterior surface of the implant. Where an anterior chamber lens shows signs of riding forwards, it may be secured by transfixing the anterior chamber with a fine needle from limbus to limbus so that the implant is kept behind the transfixing needle and away from the corneal endothelial surface (Fig. 12.4). This transfixing needle is removed at the completion of the insertion of the graft suture. When using an anterior chamber lens, it is essential that the patient has one or two patent peripheral iridectomies (Figs 12.5 and 12.6).

A posterior chamber intraocular lens using scleral support

The indication for this technique must be identified before the operation

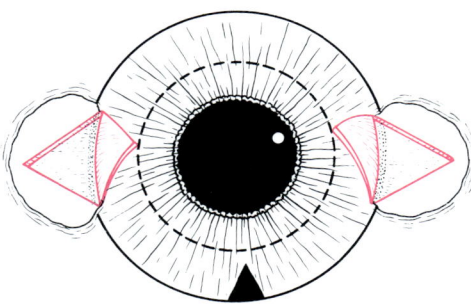

Fig. 12.7.

commences. Two small triangular, partial-thickness scleral flaps need to be raised on either side of the limbus at the 3 and 9 o'clock positions. These triangular flaps can be equilateral and have a side length of not more than 3 mm. The flaps are reflected forward to the surgical limbus. After preparation, the scleral and overlying conjunctival flaps are replaced without suturing until they are required later in the operation (Fig. 12.7).

The surgery now proceeds as for penetrating keratoplasty until the conclusion of any necessary anterior vitrectomy. A posterior-chamber-style intraocular lens, usually one piece PMMA of an appropriate power, is selected and brought into the surgical field. Using 10/0 polypropolene suture material attached to a long straight needle, approximately 14 mm in length, the end of each suture is tied to the point of the haptic at its greatest diameter (Fig. 12.8). The tie round the haptic needs to be tight enough to ensure no slippage along the haptic length. When each tie is in position, a short 28 gauge needle is passed through the centre of one of the peripheral scleral flaps, the point of the needle being directed towards the centre of the globe. The point of the needle is then rotated forwards, using the point of penetration through the sclera as a fulcrum. One of the straight needles attached to the polypropolene is now passed through the lumen of the 28 gauge needle and as soon as it has emerged, the needle through the sclera is removed. This technique minimizes uveal bleeding and allows for accurate placement of the point of fixation. The same technique is then used to place the second needle and thread.

When each needle has been passed, the intraocular implant is gently passed through the pupillary opening, and each thread in turn is then tightened to ensure that the implant takes up correct centration and without rotation. On each side, the straight needle is then passed through superficial scleral fibres in the depths of each triangular flap to produce a loop and the secure tying of the fixation knot on each side.

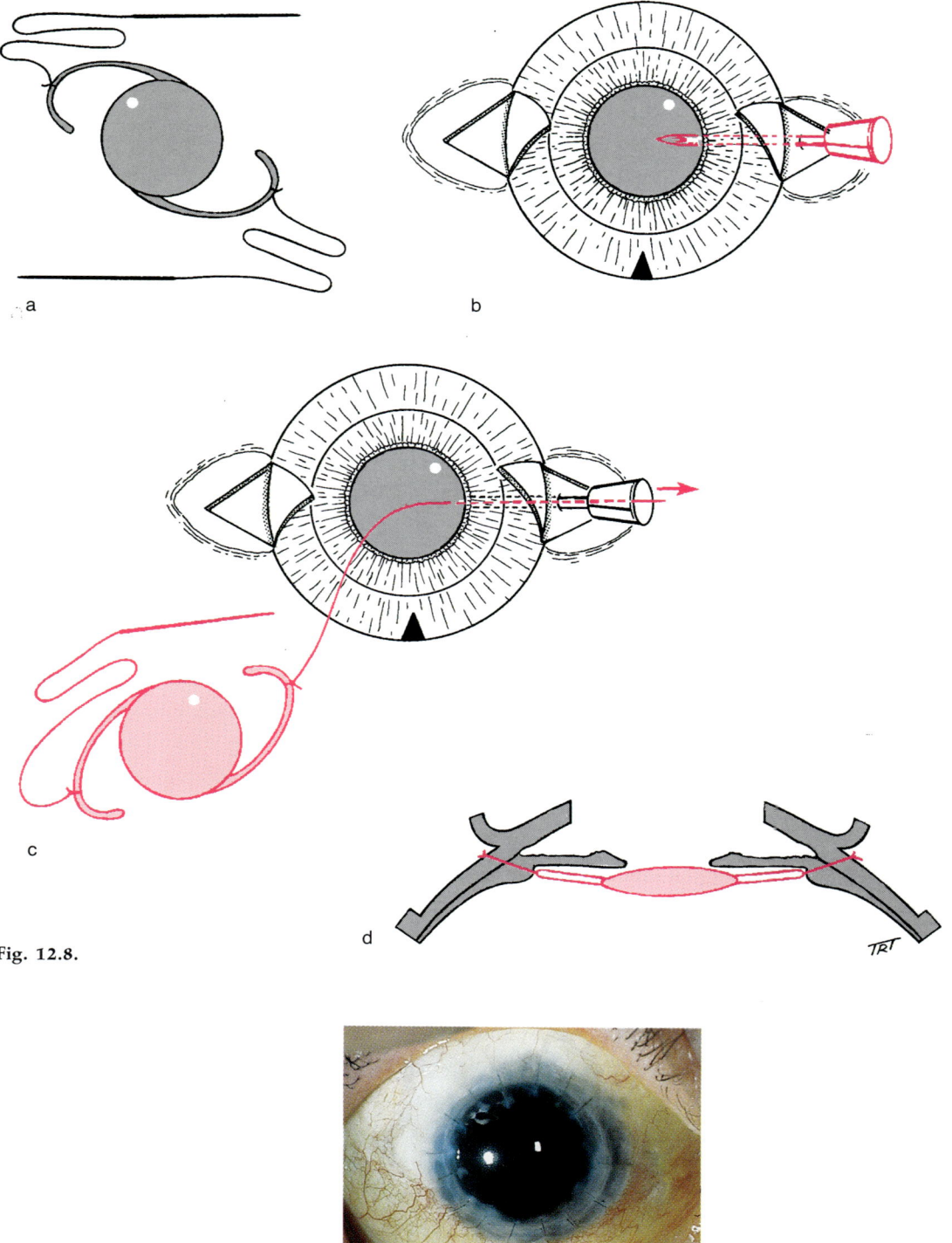

a

b

c

d

Fig. 12.8.

Fig. 12.9.

The ends are then cut short and covered by closing the scleral flaps with 10/0 nylon or 8/0 vicryl sutures. The overlying conjunctival flaps are closed using 8/0 vicryl.

The penetrating keratoplasty is now completed as for routine penetrating keratoplasty (Fig. 12.9).

13

Combined penetrating keratoplasty and glaucoma surgery

INDICATION

Corneal grafting in the presence of uncontrolled glaucoma carries a dismal prognosis. Even where the glaucoma requires topical medication for its control preoperatively, it is extremely likely that this glaucoma will become unmanageable after penetrating keratoplasty if no other measures are taken. The indication, therefore, for combined corneal and glaucoma surgery is the *presence of glaucoma which has not been controlled by surgical means previously.*

SURGICAL TECHNIQUE

1. The patient should be treated with preoperative drops of pilocarpine, as for a normal corneal graft.

2. Superior and inferior rectus sutures are inserted.

3. These sutures are now adjusted so as to expose the upper area of the limbus and adjacent conjunctiva.

4. A small, fornix-based flap is raised adjacent to the upper limbus.

5. Cautery is used to stop any bleeding and to mark out the limits of the scleral flap.

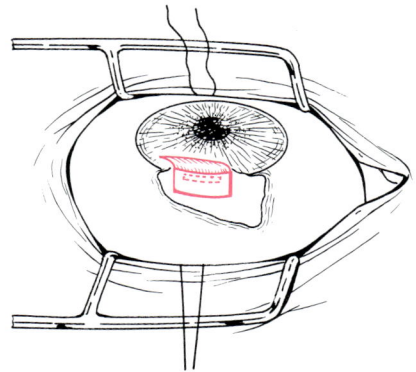

Fig. 13.1.

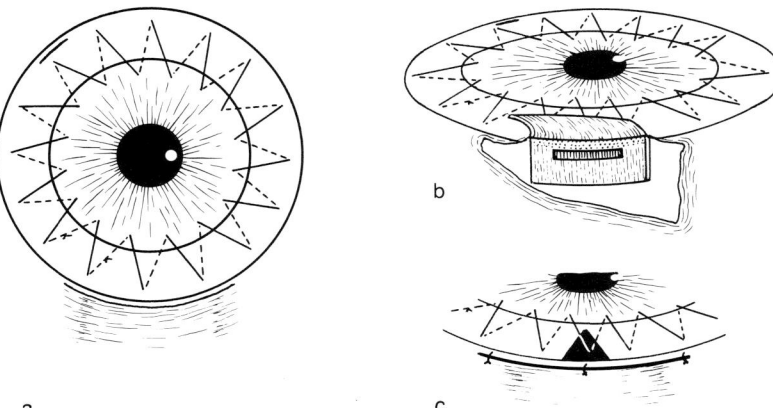

Fig. 13.2.

6. A superficial scleral flap is raised, 4 mm wide and 2–3 mm back from the limbus (Fig. 13.1). The edges should be kept sharp and clear, and the dissection should start at the back edge of the flap and be continued forward into clear cornea.

7. Using the tip of a sharp blade, the limits of the internal sclerotomy should be marked out, but care should be taken not to enter the anterior chamber at this point (Fig. 13.1).

8. The scleral and conjunctival flaps are placed back into position.

9. The superior and inferior rectus sutures are readjusted to reposition the eye so that the cornea is directed vertically upwards.

10. An anterior scleral supporting ring should be sutured into position at this stage, if it is required.

11. The usual technique for performing a corneal graft is now undertaken, and completed up to the time of finishing the knot in the continuous suture (Fig. 13.2a) or the turning in of knots of interrupted sutures into their tracks. At this stage, the anterior chamber will be formed and be of normal depth, and the corneal graft wound will be leak-free and of even contour.

12. The anterior scleral supporting ring is now removed.

13. The rectus sutures are once more readjusted so that the eye is turned to downgaze. The conjunctival and scleral flaps are retracted, and the sclerotomy is completed (Fig. 13.2b). The anterior chamber is re-deepened using visco-elastic fluid, and a small peripheral iridectomy is performed through the sclerotomy.

14. The scleral and conjunctival flaps are sutured into position using either 10/0 nylon with buried knots or 7/0 vicryl which will dissolve (Fig. 13.2c).

15. The superior and inferior rectus sutures are removed.

16. Subconjunctival injections of steroid and antibiotic solution are given in the fornices, avoiding disturbing the conjunctiva over the trabeculectomy site.

17. The eye is dressed as for a corneal graft.

18. If mitomycin C is to be used complete the dissection as far as #7 above. Mitomycin C prepared fresh by the pharmacy in a concentration of 0.4 mg/ml is used. It may be applied either soaked in a sterile cellulose sponge or in sterile filter paper. The authors prefer filter paper as the mitomycin C can then be applied to two areas more easily. The filter paper is cut to a D shape slightly larger than the scleral flap. Two pieces are made. It is soaked in the mitomycin C. One piece is applied under the flap which is then stroked back to its natural position and covered with the second piece. The conjunctiva is similarly replaced over this and the time noted. Surgeons vary in the time they apply the drug but the authors generally apply the filter paper for 3 minutes. Afterwards the paper is removed with the same forceps which are discarded. The mitomycin C must be discarded in accordance with hospital policy. The trabeculectomy site is thoroughly irrigated with a balanced salt solution taking care to irrigate under the conjunctiva and flap. The eye must not be entered prior to this point. The surgery may now continue from #8.

Silicone drainage tubing

Many of these eyes already have scarred conjunctivae, and trabeculectomy fails. Once trabeculectomy has failed we recommend the use of silicone drainage tubing to control the intraocular pressure.

The vast majority of the eyes which require this procedure are aphakic, and many will have undergone some form of vitrectomy. Such eyes are particularly prone to expulsive or delayed suprachoroidal haemorrhage when undergoing drainage surgery. In order to avoid this devastating complication, the silicone tubing should be inserted using a two-stage procedure.

Although this technique may be performed usefully for the control of postkeratoplasty glaucoma where trabeculectomy has failed or is inappropriate, it may also be combined with penetrating keratoplasty. In this case the graft should be performed at the second stage.

Stage 1

1. The conjunctiva is opened through 360° about 6–8 mm behind the

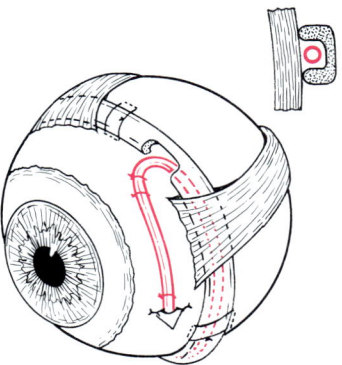

Fig. 13.3.

limbus. This reduces the tendency for the limbal conjunctiva to become ischaemic, and so lessens the subsequent risk of tube erosion. The conjunctival edges are then freed. This dissection should be done with great care, using a surgical microscope, to avoid button-holing the conjunctiva which may be followed by erosion and exposure of the tube or gutter.

2. The four recti muscles are exposed and the four quadrants are cleaned by gentle blunt dissection. A 2/0 silk sling suture may be used to isolate the recti until the gutter can be passed.

3. A standard 220 silicone gutter (used for retinal detachment surgery) is inverted so that the gutter is facing the sclera (Fig. 13.3). It is passed under the four recti, encircling the eye. Some forward planning is required at this stage, since the aim will be to insert the tube in a quadrant where the sclera is (relatively) unscathed by previous surgery. This helps to prevent tube exposure. The two free ends of the silicone gutter then need to be joined in the opposite quadrant. This helps reduce fibrosis in the region of the tube.

4. The gutter is secured in each quadrant between and behind the insertions of the recti muscles with 5/0 Ethibond mattress sutures. The gutter should not indent the globe; it only has to be firmly secured. The free ends are trimmed so the gutter is snug, neither too loose nor too tight, and the ends are sutured together with 5/0 Ethibond.

5. The drainage tube itself is 0.63-mm external bore silicone tubing. In the quadrant where the tube will enter the eye, a small section is cut out of the gutter so that the tube can be placed into the gutter without being compressed by the side. One end is passed under the gutter through about 90°. It is secured to the sclera and the gutter by two tight (but not constricting) 9/0 nylon sutures. Alternatively,

the tube can be prepared earlier by gluing the tube to the gutter with silicone glue. The whole 'ensemble' must then be sterilized.

A long free end is left. This is tucked under the nearest rectus muscle, and the free end buried in a small, triangular, partial-thickness flap of sclera, secured with nylon. This will help to identify the free end later, and prevent excessive fibrosis within the tube (Fig. 13.3).

6. If it is felt that the intraocular pressure is so high that the optic disc will be compromised before the second stage, a trabeculectomy with a well-sutured flap can be performed at a site distant from the tube.

7. The conjunctiva is then very carefully closed with 8/0 virgin silk or polyglycolate. An accurate diagram of the position of the tube and gutter should be made in the clinical notes to ease identification at the next stage.

8. A subconjunctival injection of antibiotic and steroid should be given at this stage.

Postoperative care

Topical antibiotics and steroids, and any antiglaucoma medication that may be necessary should be continued until the second stage.

In some circumstances (e.g. where there is extensive conjunctival scarring or a previous failed graft) it may be appropriate to combine trabeculectomy with intraoperative *mitomycin C*. For discussion of this technique see above, p. 76, number 18.

Stage 2

1. The second stage can be performed 4–8 weeks later. In that time, a fibrovascular sheath forms around the gutter. This will provide resistance to the outflow of aqueous when the tube is inserted. It is also responsible for absorbing the aqueous.

2. The conjunctiva is opened only in the quadrant where the tube will be inserted and over the free end of the tube, and carefully reflected.

3. A wide scleral flap is raised (rather as one might for trabeculectomy), at least 6 mm wide and extending up to the gutter. It should be as deep as possible – ideally at least 7/8ths the depth of the sclera. This flap should be raised as far forward as the grey line at the limbus (Fig. 13.4). When a penetrating graft is to be performed as part of the procedure, it is done at this point.

4. The free end of the tube is trimmed so that approximately 4 mm will protrude into the anterior chamber. Its patency is checked by

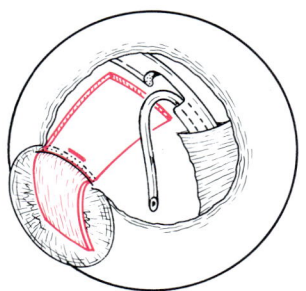

Fig. 13.4.

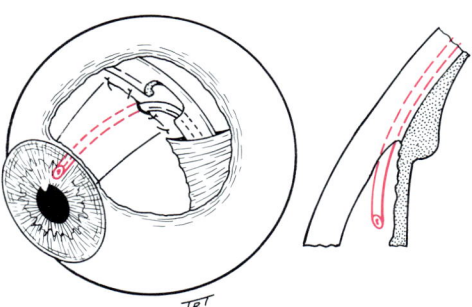

Fig. 13.5.

flushing through with balanced salt solution with a Rycroft cannula. It is fixed to the sclera under the flap by a 9/0 nylon suture, and the anterior chamber is penetrated by a 25 gauge needle or knife.

5. The tube is inserted into the anterior chamber through this puncture, and the scleral flap secured with 9/0 nylon (Fig. 13.5).

6. The conjunctiva is closed carefully, and an orbital floor injection of steroid may be given.

7. A subconjunctival injection should be avoided in case of inadvertent reverse flow through the tube, and injection into the eye.

8. If there is significant residual vitreous gel, it must be removed before the tube is inserted; otherwise, drainage of fluid will tend to suck the gel into the tube, causing blockage. This may be done through the standard pars plana approach either at the first or the second stage.

It is important to conform with hospital regulations concerning the disposal of powerful antimetabolites such as mitomycin C.

Postoperative care

The patient requires topical antibiotic drops until the eye has healed, and topical dexamethasone 0.1% or prednisolone 1% drops six times a day permanently. If this regimen is not used the patient is exposed to risk of graft rejection, and this surgery will have been in vain (Fig. 13.6).

Complications

1. Tube blockage with vitreous can occur if an inadequate vitrectomy has been performed. This may also happen if there was not a posterior vitreous detachment (PVD) at the time of surgery, and the cortical gel was left in situ. Subsequent PVD with forward displacement can lead to blockage of the tube. Laser disruption can be attempted but is rarely successful, and a vitrectomy will be

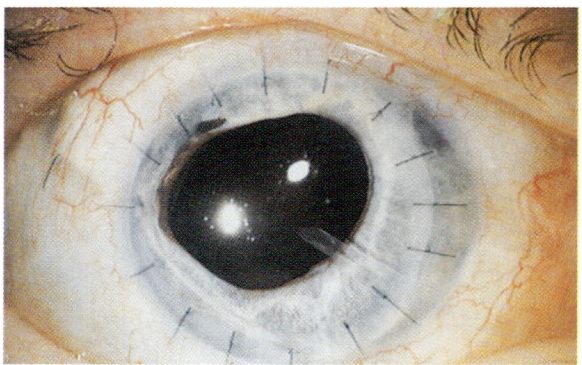

Fig. 13.6

necessary. Patency of the tube should be checked at the end of the procedure.

2. Despite even the most careful dissection, the tube may erode through the conjunctiva, predisposing the eye to endophthalmitis. If this happens, the conjunctiva may be repaired, but usually by this stage it will be too thin for security. In this situation, it is worthwhile covering the tube with a scleral patch graft from a donor eye, and covering this with a free conjunctival graft from the contralateral eye.

3. Delayed choroidal haemorrhage may occur even after a two-stage procedure. The results are disappointing, but it may be worthwhile draining the choroidal haemorrhage through a full thickness scleral incision over the haemorrhage, and restoring the eye to normal pressure with injection of C_2F_6 gas. Once the haemorrhage has been drained as fully as possible, the tube should be ligated and the pressure restored to normality with further gas. The sclera can be sutured with 8/0 nylon.

4. If endophthalmitis does occur, it must be treated in the usual fashion with vitreous biopsy or vitrectomy and injection of appropriate intravitreal antibiotics.

The diode laser
Developed since the first edition of this manual, this device has been found to be a useful addition to the management of some cases of otherwise intractable glaucoma.

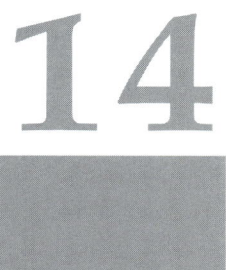

Early postoperative complications

WOUND LEAKAGE

Wound leakage will be detected by a fall in intraocular pressure and a positive Seidel's test. The patient will need to be taken back to the operating theatre, and further interrupted sutures added to the wound to stop the leakage (Fig. 14.1).

DELAYED EPITHELIALIZATION (Fig. 14.2)

Occasionally, where a stored disc has no secure epithelium, a large epithelial defect will persist for several days after corneal grafting. During this period, the patient should be kept under regular observation, as there is greater risk of infection during this period. Intensive drop medication can aggravate the problem and delay epithelialization. Padding the eye, or taping the lid is often the best solution. Very large grafts can pose a particular problem. In any case where there is no sign of useful healing of large epithelial defects, consideration may be given for a botulinum toxin protective ptosis (see Ch. 19).

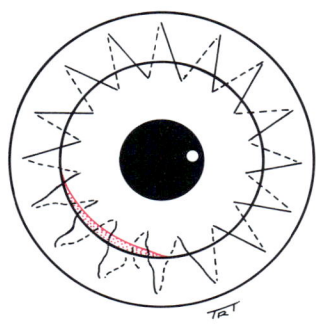

Fig. 14.1.

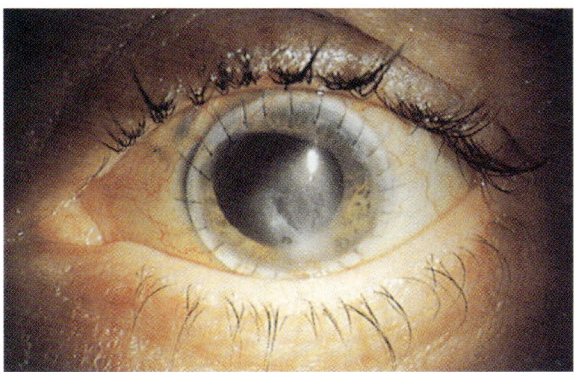

Fig. 14.2.

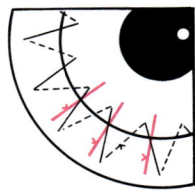

Fig. 14.3.

INFECTION

Early infection is rare, but infrequent cases of endophthalmitis may be encountered. Sudden onset of pain, loss of vision and discharge associated with flare, cells, fibrin or hypopyon, vitreous opacity, retinal vascular sheathing and a relative afferent pupillary defect demand urgent investigation. Prompt vitreous biopsy and intravitreal antibiotics may be sight-saving. Suture-related infections and microbial infections are more likely to be late complications (see Ch. 15).

EARLY SUTURE PROBLEMS

As indicated above, some patients are at risk of early suture-loosening, particularly children or patients who have had preoperative vascularization of the host stroma or whose operation has been performed while the eye has been inflamed. Loose sutures must always be removed immediately. Where this gives rise to insecurity of the wound, further interrupted sutures must be added. In vascularized areas, however, the corneal graft wound will be likely to have healed early so that further suturing may not be necessary.

Where a segment of continuous suture has loosened in the early postoperative period, there is doubt as to the integrity of the wound. Resuturing should not be postponed. Usually, even a running suture that has loosened should be replaced with interrupted sutures (Fig. 14.3).

UVEITIS

Postoperatively, patients need to be treated with sufficient local steroid to suppress signs of uveitis. Should uveitis reassert itself after its original postoperative suppression, the surgeon should suspect the re-emergence of a viral inflammation, in appropriate cases, or an early graft rejection process.

GLAUCOMA

After corneal grafting, the intraocular pressure must be measured at every postoperative attendance. This is because grafting can alter the profile of the anterior chamber of the eye and possibly interfere with normal filtration, and also because patients are using steroid medication for some months. This, of course, can always be associated with a rise in intraocular pressure. Post-keratoplasty glaucoma may have an incidence as high as 30–50% in some aphakic and pseudophakic eyes. Its early detection is essential. Glaucoma may be managed by adjustment of the steroid dosage, or topical and systemic glaucoma therapy. Occasionally, filtration surgery will be required.

CATARACT

The development of a cataract in the postoperative period after corneal grafting may be due to a failure to diagnose pre-existing cataract, or to damage to the lens surface at the time of corneal grafting or to the development of posterior subcapsular lens opacities associated with high levels of steroid medication. When the cataract develops to such a degree that it is interfering with the patient's good vision, extracapsular cataract extraction and the insertion of a posterior chamber intraocular lens will need to be undertaken. Where possible this should be delayed until at least 6 months after keratoplasty, to reduce the risk of trauma to the new graft and to avoid precipitating a rejection episode.

PRIMARY GRAFT FAILURE

Occasionally, the corneal graft will fail to clear postoperatively, and gross oedema will persist despite high levels of topical medication. If there is no sign of disc endothelial function at the end of one week, a primary graft failure should be presumed and arrangements made for replacement of the donor disc with a healthy substitute. Serial pachometry may help to monitor endothelial function.

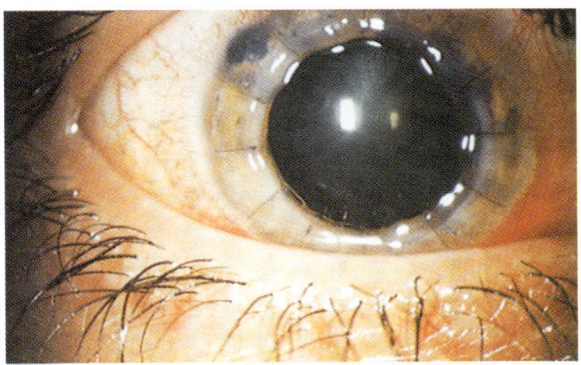

Fig. 14.4.

URRETS–ZAVALIA SYNDROME

The Urrets–Zavalia syndrome, characterized by a widely and irreversibly dilated pupil, may be found after any type of penetrating graft. It is due to ischaemia of the sphincter pupillae, which is most likely to have occurred perioperatively due to high vitreous pressure pushing the lens forward, compressing the iris against the peripheral host cornea. There is no treatment but good anaesthesia and avoidance of needlessly prolonged procedures should help to avoid the problem (Fig. 14.4).

Late postoperative complications

SUTURE PROBLEMS

Sutures may loosen at any time after corneal grafting and are a hazard for the corneal graft, giving rise to surface irritation, vascularization and the risk of infection and rejection. They must always be removed promptly. In the late postoperative period, there is little to be gained from trimming loose loops and the whole suture should be removed. If there is doubt as to the integrity of the wound, resuturing may be required (Fig. 15.1).

GRAFT REJECTION

Any corneal graft, other than an autograft, can reject at any time, even after many years. Regrafts may reject early, but first grafts rarely reject before 10 days. Patients must be warned that soreness, redness or misting of vision must be reported to their ophthalmologist without delay. Signs of corneal graft rejection include: limbal injection; flare and cells with (Fig. 15.2) or without precipitates; an endothelial rejection line; stromal and epithelial oedema behind the rejection line (Fig. 15.3); an epithelial rejection line; Krachmer's spots (Fig. 15.4) and loss of vision if corneal oedema includes the visual axis.

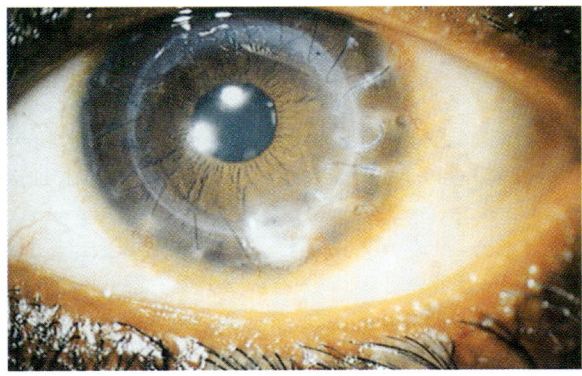

Fig. 15.1.

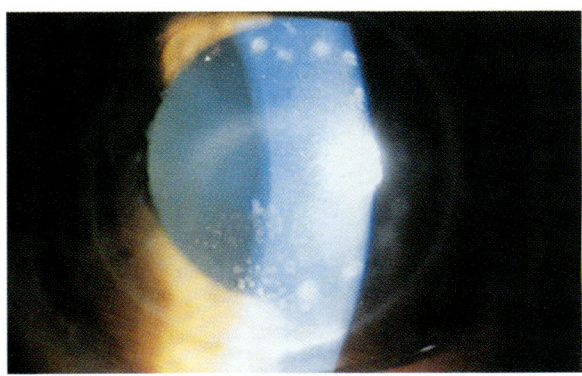

Fig. 15.2.

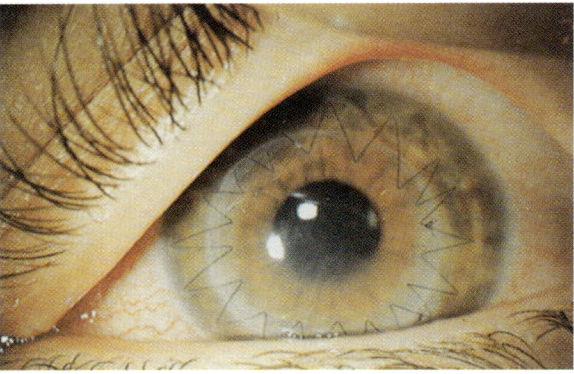

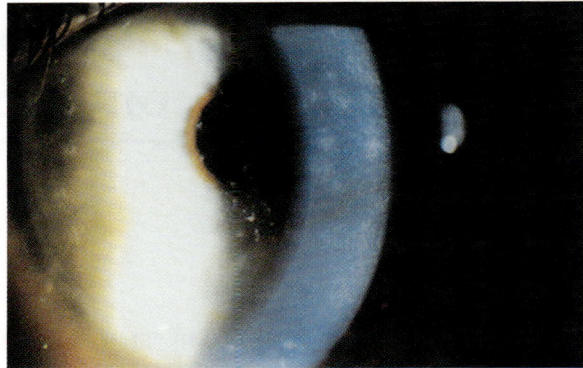

Fig. 15.3.   Fig. 15.4.

Epithelial rejection on its own may not be a hazard to the corneal graft, but should be treated aggressively as it may rapidly be followed by endothelial rejection which, of course, is potentially much more damaging. Graft rejection is best treated by admission to hospital for intensive round-the-clock medication, with daily injections of soluble steroid and topical dexamethasone (or similar preparation), half-hourly throughout the 24-hour period. This level of medication may be required for three or four days in order to achieve a reversal of the rejection. There is increasing evidence that an intravenous single pulse of methylprednisolone may also be beneficial in difficult rejections. A dose of 500–1000 mg depending on body weight given over a 30-minute period is used.

VASCULARIZATION

Host stroma will usually only vascularize after corneal grafting if there is irritation of the corneal surface or some other cause for persistent inflammation. Corneal graft sutures should not, therefore, be placed closer to the limbus than is absolutely necessary in order to achieve wound security. Having said this, however, sutures which do include or even cross the limbus do not usually give rise to the ingrowth of vessels. In most cases treatment is not necessary but occasionally lipid keratopathy may develop and argon laser of the vessels may be helpful. The feeder arteriole must be identifiable. It is occluded with minimum necessary power and spot size between limbus and graft–host interface. Several attempts may be necessary as fresh feeders may open up.

GLAUCOMA

As stated in Chapter 14, it is essential to keep a watch on the possible late onset of post-keratoplasty glaucoma. Although this book is primarily surgical, the authors would note that an additional modality has been introduced into the treatment of difficult glaucomas. The diode laser may be used to deliver very precise laser burns to the ciliary body. This is much more controlled than either cyclocryoablation or cyclo-YAG-ablation. The procedure can be performed under local anaesthesia at the slit lamp or under the operating microscope. Approximately 15 burns are made over the ciliary body avoiding the 3 and 9 o'clock meridians to avoid damage to the long ciliary nerves. The procedure is repeatable and offers a good prospect of IOP control. It should be noted that post-keratoplasty glaucoma has not been specifically studied with this treatment but initial reports are encouraging.

CATARACT

See Chapter 14.

LATE WOUND FAILURE

Corneal graft sutures are usually left in place for 12 months. Patients who then enjoy good vision with the suture in place should be left alone, but for others the suture is usually removed. Occasionally, this process may be followed by the development of a step in the wound profile, due to inadequate healing and wound slippage. This needs to be detected early, and usually requires resuturing of the wound in order to restore proper curvature as well as anticipating complete wound rupture. Failure to do this will certainly give rise to post-graft astigmatism of a high degree, and will eventually require treatment (see Ch. 21). Graft wounds are also susceptible to rupture after relatively minor blunt trauma even many years after surgery.

RECURRENCE OF A PRE-EXISTING DISORDER

Many corneal grafts are done for a variety of corneal dystrophies and also for scarring due to viral disease, particularly herpes simplex. These conditions are liable to recur and patients need to be warned that this is the case.

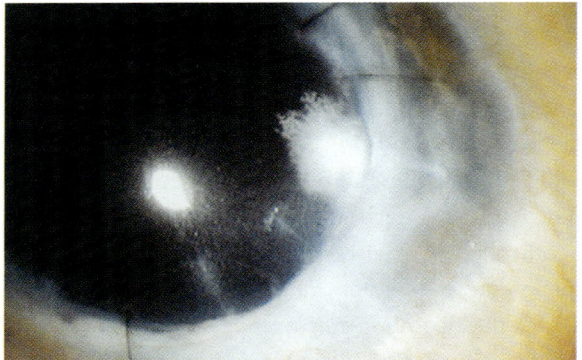

Fig. 15.5.

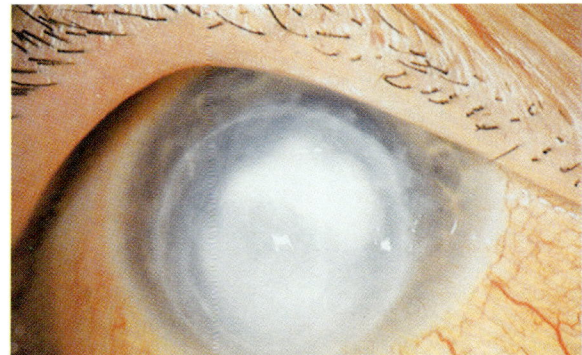

Fig. 15.6.

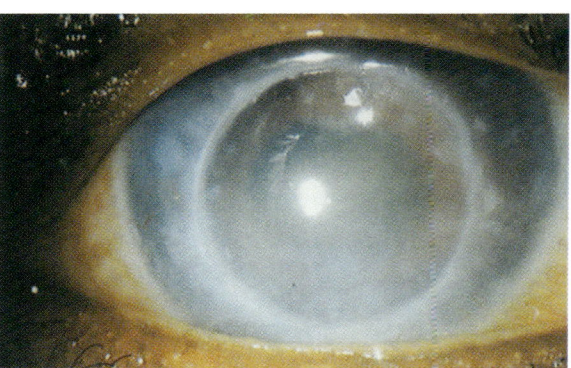

Fig. 15.7.

ASTIGMATISM (See Ch. 20)

MICROBIAL KERATITIS

This may be encountered in as many as one in 30 grafts, but risk factors include loose sutures (Fig. 15.5), ocular surface disease (Fig 15.6) and an established graft failure (Fig. 15.7). Corneal scrape for microscopy and culture is essential, as is appropriate topical antibiotic therapy. Broad spectrum therapy, with gentamicin 1.5% drops and cefuroxime 5% drops alternating every 15 minutes, may be started in anticipation of laboratory results. Depending upon the clinical response microscopy, culture and sensitivity results may permit modification of this regimen. For cases of crystalline keratopathy, a biopsy (see Ch. 6) may be necessary.

ENDOTHELIAL DECOMPENSATION AND FAILURE OF THE GRAFT

Any one of the above complications may lead to irreversible endothelial decompensation and failure of the graft (Fig. 15.7). Every effort should be made to avoid this complication, as regrafting carries a much worse prognosis since it carries a higher risk of complications and graft failure, particularly for those grafts which fail due to immunological factors.

16

Emergency penetrating keratoplasty

Spontaneous perforations (or incipient perforations) too large for glue (see Ch. 19) may occur in the course of a number of conditions, such as microbial keratitis, rheumatoid corneal melt, either central or peripheral, herpes simplex keratitis, or Mooren's ulceration. When this happens, emergency keratoplasty is required to save the eye and, hopefully, restore vision. The authors do not recommend delay for any reason other than unavailability of donor material or severe associated systemic problems which preclude surgery.

In some corneal infections, uncontrolled by medication, scleral invasion may occur or be threatened. Keratoplasty may be indicated as the only way open to control the infective process.

In cases where the perforation is sterile and small, some authorities recommend a lamellar onlay graft. The present authors do not favour this approach.

SURGICAL TECHNIQUE

The basic techniques of keratoplasty are applied but certain modifications are useful. If the perforation is small and is not in necrotic tissue, it may be possible to apply cyanoacrylate glue on the perforation before trephining the graft. This can be particularly useful, though time consuming, since it may allow the anterior chamber to be restored with visco-elastic and the trephination can then be done on an eye with relatively normal intraocular pressure. For less experienced surgeons (and often this type of surgery has to be done by the less experienced), it may even be helpful for a larger perforation to be sealed temporarily until the graft can be trephined. This may be achieved by cutting a patch from a hydrogel lens, gluing this patch in situ with 'superglue' and once dry in a few minutes restoring the anterior chamber and proceeding to keratoplasty. We must emphasize that this is a temporary measure, and must not be used as a long-term solution.

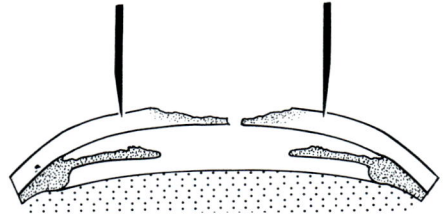

Fig. 16.1.

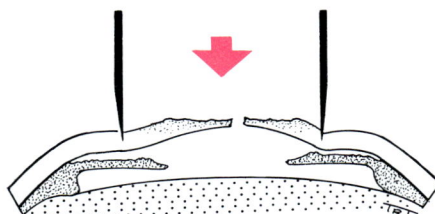

Fig. 16.2.

1. If the eye is aphakic, the usual precaution of a scleral supporting ring may have to be avoided, as the manipulation involved may cause further prolapse of the intraocular contents. For the same reason, rectus fixation should also be avoided.

2. It is important that the wound be made in healthy tissue even if this means that the wound has to extend beyond the limbus, in which case a peritomy will be necessary.

3. The probable extent of the graft should be measured, and a trephine large enough to include all affected tissue should be chosen and the cornea lightly marked (Fig. 16.1).

4. At all times, undue pressure on the globe should be avoided to prevent extrusion of the intraocular contents (Fig. 16.2). This is especially important when trephining as the soft perforated eye reacts very differently to trephination.

5. The trephine mark can then be deepened freehand with a sharp blade.

6. The cord length of this mark should be carefully measured.

7. Once the extent of the host bed has been clearly defined, the donor tissue may be dissected.

8. If the graft has to be so large as to include the limbus, there may be problems with re-epithelialization. If possible, a slightly eccentric graft should be performed so that some healthy host limbus remains (Fig. 16.3). Alternatively, it may be possible to perform a sector keratoplasty (Figs 16.4 and 16.5).

9. It is important that the donor disc should be large enough to fill the host bed, and the cord length of the donor should be accurately compared with that measured on the host. Account should be taken of any collapse of the host anterior chamber and any consequent distortion. It is often necessary to cut a donor disc 0.5 or 1 mm larger than the host bed. The use of a whole donor eye allows considerable flexibility at this point, but if a punch must be used for

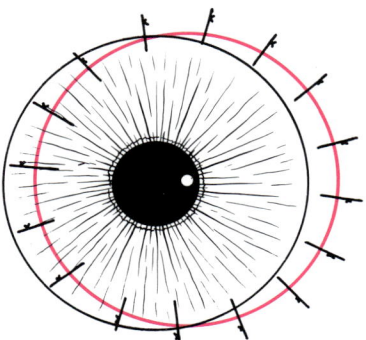

Fig. 16.3.

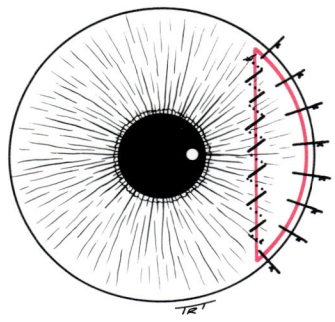

Fig. 16.4.

a corneoscleral disc, then it is best to err on the side of oversizing the donor. It can always be trimmed later. A whole eye may also have intact epithelium, which will help in the immediate post-operative period, although in most corneas stored in tissue support medium, the epithelium is usually healthy.

10. The host tissue can now be dissected. The groove made by the trephine should be gradually deepened (Fig. 16.6) using a diamond knife.

11. Once the anterior chamber has been entered, copious use should be made of visco-elastic substances. In this situation, sodium hyaluronate is preferable. This helps in a twofold fashion. Firstly, it deepens the anterior chamber and prevents damage to the underlying tissues when completing the dissection, with graft scissors or the diamond blade. Secondly, visco-elastic delamination will help to open the angle and may reduce the risk of closed-angle glaucoma (Fig. 16.7).

12. If, as is likely, there is a cyclitic membrane in the anterior chamber,

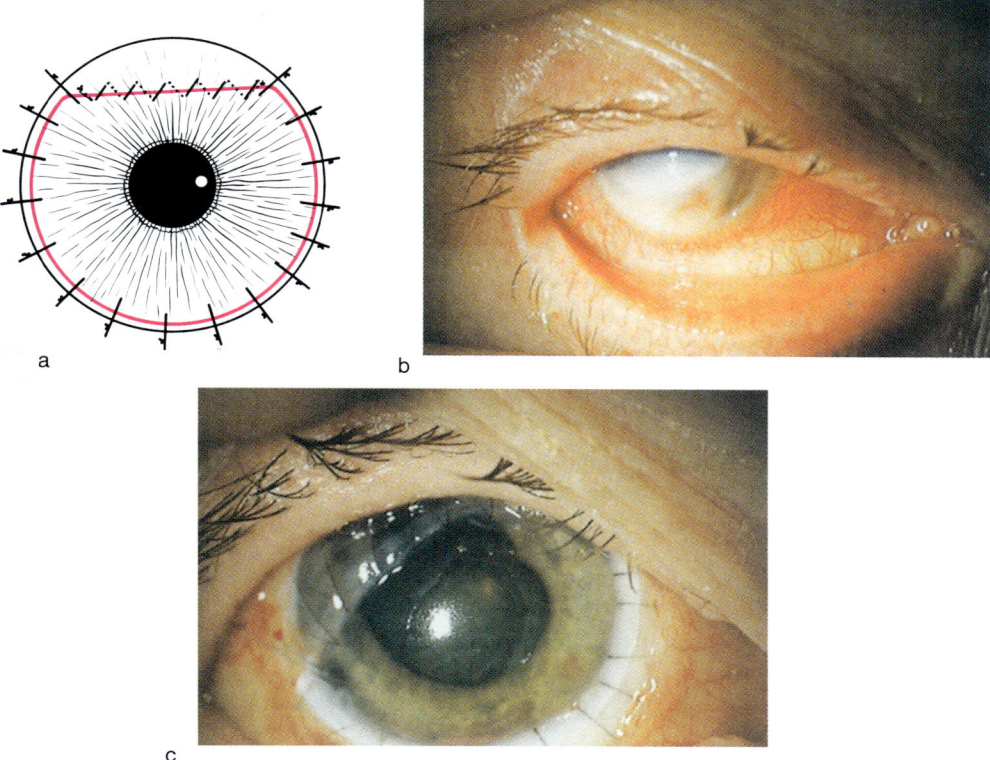

Fig. 16.5.

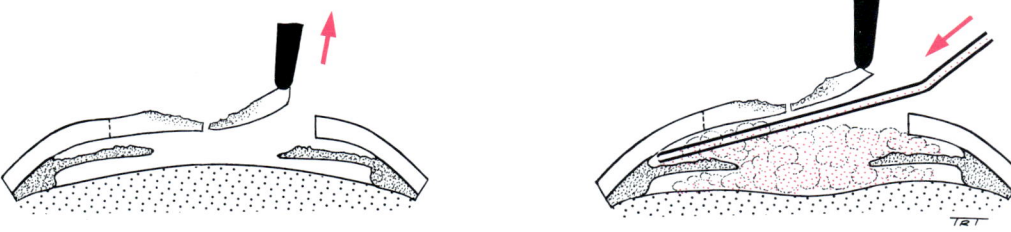

Fig. 16.6.   Fig. 16.7.

it, and any other inflammatory debris should be removed to help reduce postoperative inflammation. A peripheral iridectomy will help to prevent iris bombé in the postoperative period.

13. Removal of the crystalline lens should be avoided at this time, unless it is intumescent, subluxed or involved in the inflammatory or infective process. If the eye is already aphakic, open sky vitrectomy may speed recovery by removing inflammatory debris, but may also prevent vitreous incarceration in the wound.

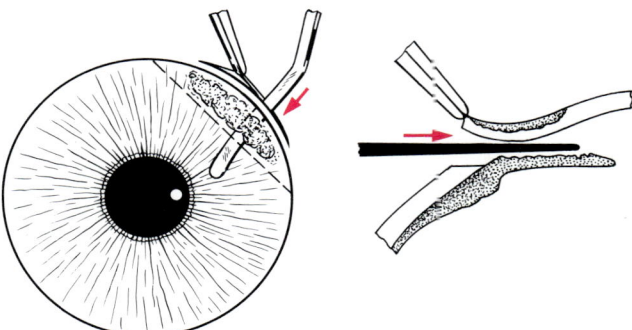

Fig. 16.8.

14. If the wound has extended beyond the limbus, care in dissection is important to avoid injury to the ciliary body. Once the incision has been completed, the scleral spur can be gently disinserted by blunt dissection with an iris repositor or cyclodialysis spatula (Fig. 16.8).

15. If sector keratoplasty is attempted, the host should be prepared and the maximum cord length measured. A circular donor disc large enough to fit this can then be cut. The host bed is prepared as above, but the straight segment has to be cut freehand. The donor is then sutured in place, until the curved portion is secure. At this point, the excess sector must be excised and a straight edge formed. Again, this is done freehand with a blade or straight scissors. Watertight closure is achieved by using a running suture along the straight edge. In some cases, e.g. rheumatoid peripheral corneal guttering, it may be preferable to insert a patch graft as shown in Figure 16.9. A peritomy will be necessary (Fig. 16.10). Two trephines of appropriate size are chosen to mark just beyond the inner and outer margins of the gutter (Fig. 16.11 and 16.12). The trephines should be applied concentrically. The distance between the two marks is carefully measured and noted (this distance must be at least as great in the donor). The two grooves are deepened and a freehand straight groove made in healthy tissue at either end

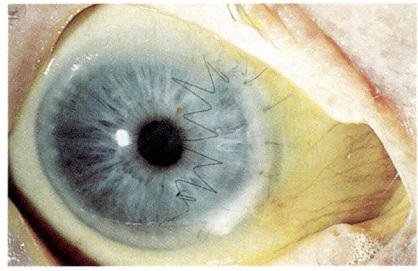

Fig. 16.9.

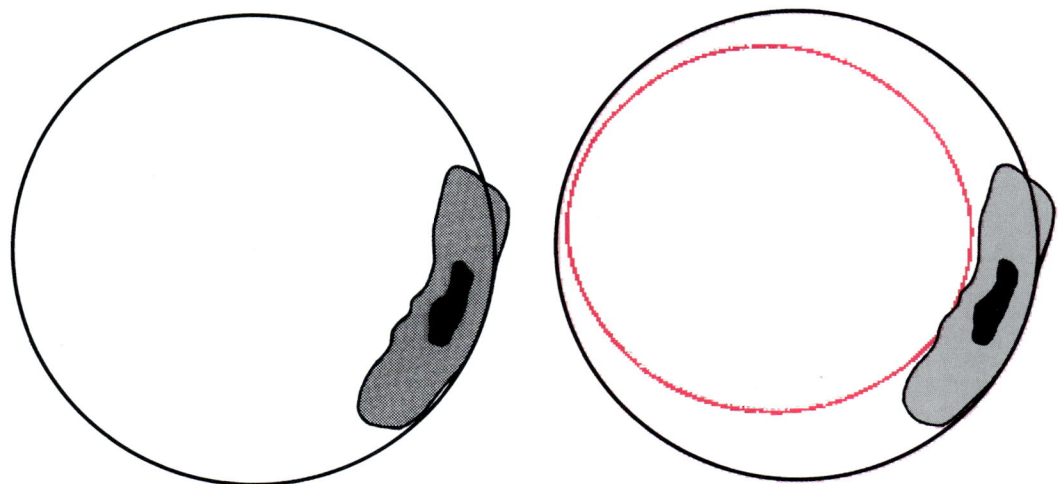

Fig. 16.10.

Fig. 16.11.

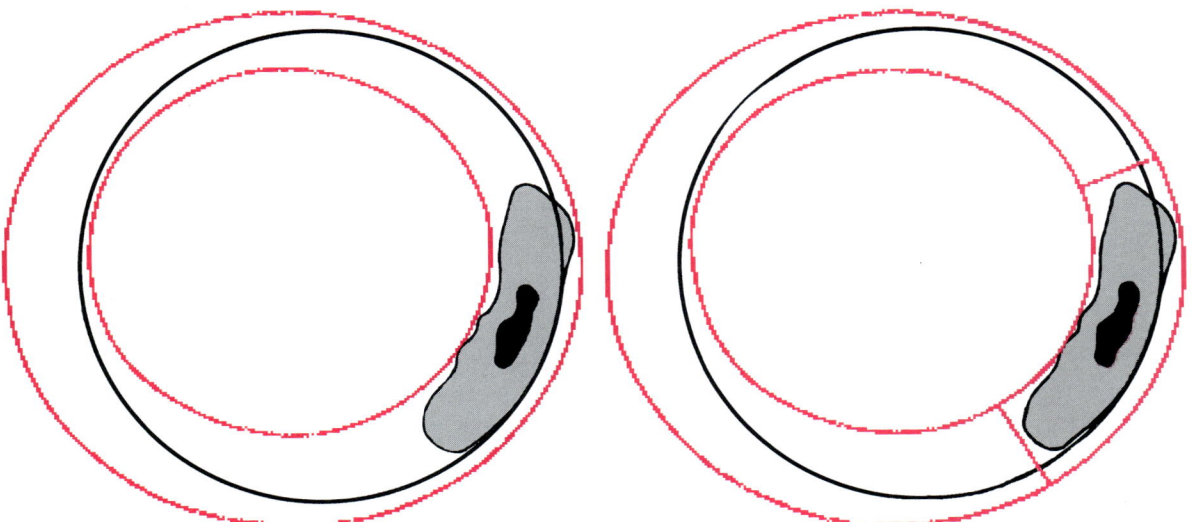

Fig. 16.12.

Fig. 16.13.

of the gutter (Fig 16.13). Essentially, the same process is repeated on the donor for which a whole eye is essential. It is wise not to truncate the patch at this stage as excess tissue can be trimmed off once the patch is inserted into the host bed. It is essential to ensure that the patch is wide enough to fit into the host bed particularly if there has been some collapse of the anterior chamber. It may be easier to achieve a watertight closure if a running suture is used. Additional interrupted sutures may be necessary.

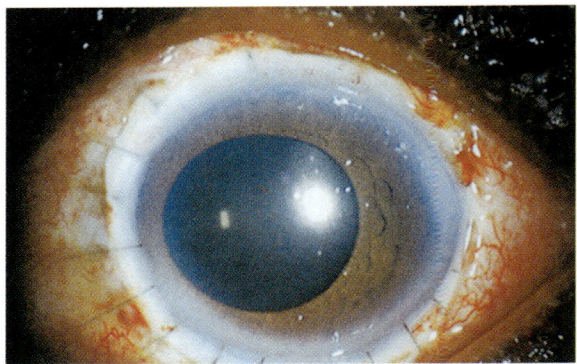

Fig. 16.14.

16. Whatever suturing pattern the surgeon normally uses, with the exceptions just discussed, interrupted sutures are advisable. There is a good chance of cheese-wiring, and if this happens a single loose suture can easily be removed. If a continuous stitch has been used, resuturing will almost certainly be necessary. Long deep bites of the 10/0 nylon, which should not be overtight, will give the best chance of stability. Enough sutures to secure the donor in good position and achieve a watertight wound should be inserted. There is no need to put in extra sutures 'just for good measure'. Too many stitches are as bad as too few.

17. The anterior chamber should be retained with visco-elastic fluid. This will not only protect the donor endothelium but will also help to tamponade any bleeding from the scleral edge, iris or angle.

18. If a corneoscleral graft has been necessary, the bare sclera should be covered with host conjunctiva sutured with 8/0 virgin silk (Fig. 16.14).

19. For infected cases, samples of all excised tissue should be sent for microbiology as well as for histological examination.

20. Appropriate antibiotics should be given by injection subconjunctivally, and subconjunctival betamethasone should also be given, even if the infecting agent was Pseudomonas or a fungus, on the basis that all the infected tissue has been eradicated. Where there is a choice of antibiotic the least toxic to the corneal epithelial and endothelial surfaces should be used.

POSTOPERATIVE CARE

These grafts are at considerable risk of rejection and will require high-dose topical steroids for a prolonged period postoperatively. If the graft has been very large (e.g. > 10 mm) then topical steroids may have to be continued indefinitely. The topical antibiotic therapy should be continued until it is clear that there is no continuing infection and should be modified where necessary by laboratory evidence. Depending on the circumstances, systemic immune suppression may also be required not just to prevent graft rejection but also to control an underlying disease process.

COMPLICATIONS

Complications are common after this procedure. Most can be treated according to general principles (see above). Glaucoma is relatively common and more likely to be severe the longer the eye has been perforated, due to inevitable angle closure. Medical therapy, followed by augmented trabeculectomy and, ultimately, silicone drainage tubing should be used whenever necessary. The diode laser can also have a useful role in the management of intractable glaucoma.

Cataract is also a common sequela, but this should not tempt the surgeon to contemplate a combined extraction with the graft. This creates more problems than it will solve. Conventional cataract surgery can be undertaken after 6 months with minimal risk to the graft and good prospects of visual recovery. Only if the cataract becomes hypermature should extraction be considered earlier.

One of the most troublesome complications is the development of further infective episodes. It is worth remembering that many of these eyes perforate or become infected because of ocular surface disease, and they remain at risk after keratoplasty. Such patients need careful postoperative supervision and prompt investigation of any suspected recurrence.

Large grafts involving the limbus may be very slow to re-epithelialize, and botulinum toxin protective ptosis may be required (see Ch. 19). There is some anecdotal evidence that the use of an eccentrically cut donor, which includes limbal stem cells, may help epithelialization. Such a situation probably requires systemic immune suppression.

Section C
Lamellar techniques

17

Lamellar keratoplasty

The indications for lamellar keratoplasty are varied, but in general they include conditions where the anterior cornea is opaque and where there is healthy stroma behind the opacity, combined with a healthy endothelium. Lamellar keratoplasty may also have to be combined with excision of a recurrent pterygium if the previous surgery has led to marked loss of tissue. Just as penetrating keratoplasty is often contra-indicated in cases of severe ocular surface abnormality, so also is lamellar keratoplasty. The advantage of lamellar keratoplasty is that it is repeatable several times and there is no risk of endothelial rejection although, of course, stromal epithelial rejection may occur.

The procedure is usually prolonged and delicate, and for this reason is best done under general anaesthesia. The usual instruments for keratoplasty are required but, in addition, a range of lamellar dissectors is available.

DONOR

Since perforation can occur even in the most skilled hands, a donor suitable for penetrating keratoplasty should be available; however, the requirements for a donor for lamellar keratoplasty alone are much less stringent. Providing that the eye has been stored in a moist chamber at 4°C, and that the postmortem to enucleation time was not too long, the stroma should be usable up to 7 days postmortem. After this length of time, however, the tissue is very oedematous and dissection very difficult. A recently enucleated eye is as difficult to dissect as the host. A small amount of oedema in the stroma, however, allows the lamellae to be split more easily. A whole eye is almost essential for a lamellar keratoplasty, and the authors would suggest that anyone inexperienced in performing a lamellar graft should not attempt a lamellar dissection on a stored corneoscleral disc.

In most instances, the lamellar graft needs to be at least half the thickness of the stroma, but in many situations the dissection is carried

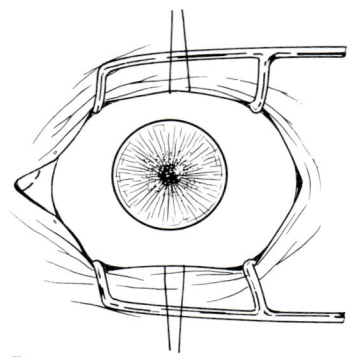

Fig. 17.1.

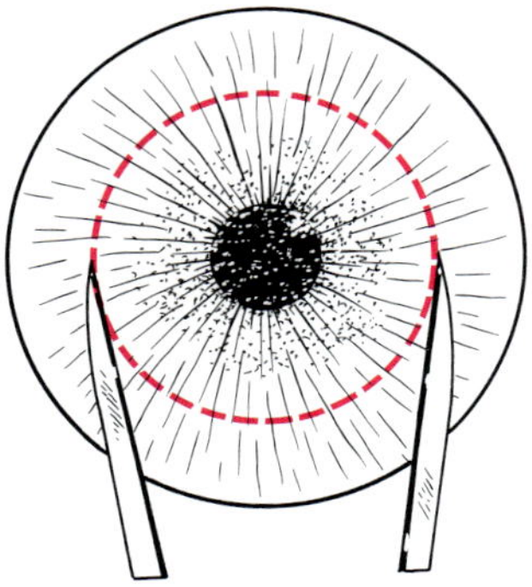

Fig. 17.2.

Fig. 17.3.

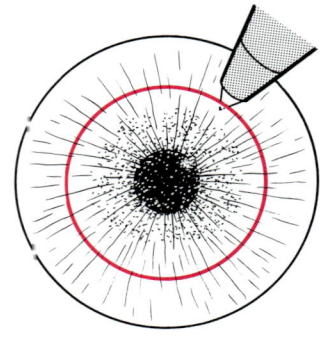

down to Descemet's membrane. In these cases only is it then possible to use a full thickness donor disc cut from a stored corneoscleral button.

SURGICAL TECHNIQUE

1. The eye is stabilized with superior and inferior rectus fixation sutures (Fig. 17.1).

2. The extent of the graft is marked with a trephine, and the wound edge is deepened. This is best done under direct visual control since perforation of the eye is to be avoided at all costs. If the eye is perforated, then the procedure usually needs to be converted to a penetrating keratoplasty. For this reason, the graft should never be larger than necessary. It is difficult to cut the whole wound edge to a uniform depth, but this is less important.

3. The cord length of this mark should be carefully measured (Fig. 17.2).

4. At the point nearest the surgeon, the wound should extend as deeply as has been estimated to be necessary. This deepening may have to be done very cautiously, a few lamellae at a time (Fig. 17.3).

5. Once the desired depth is reached, the lamellae are split gently using a Paufique knife, forming a little pocket in the stroma (Fig. 17.4).

6. As the pocket enlarges, superficial lamellae remaining uncut at the wound edge are divided by an upcut with a diamond blade so that a disc of cornea is slowly released (Fig. 17.5). The dissection is gradually extended, always staying within the same lamella.

7. As one passes over 'the brow of the hill' of the cornea, the dissection is made easier by the variety of dissectors, but by no means all are essential. The more lamellae that are cut, the greater

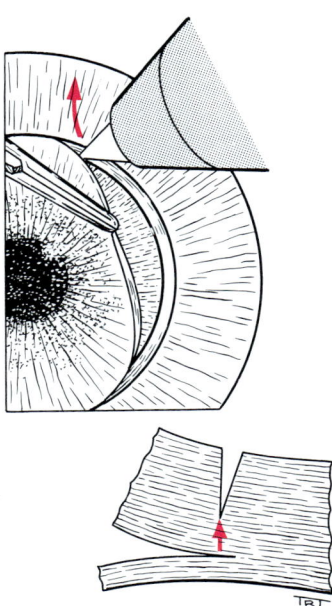

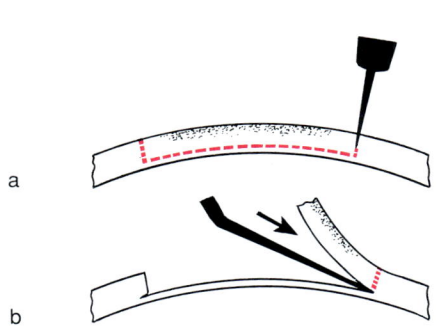

Fig. 17.4.   **Fig. 17.5.**

the interface opacity that will ensue, reducing the final acuity. Gentle, patient and painstaking dissection will be rewarded with a much smoother surface. The dissection is essentially blunt, with the lamellae being split apart. Sharp instruments risk perforation, but may be required at the edge of the host bed. Here, the cut is made upwards always to avoid dissection (Fig. 17.5).

8. Having successfully dissected the host, the donor is prepared. The donor eye should be prepared in the same way as for a penetrating keratoplasty. While this is being done, the host cornea should be covered with a moist swab.

9. The globe can be supported in an eye stand, preferably one which allows control of the intraocular pressure.

10. If the epithelium is loose, it should be removed with a cellulose swab.

11. The trephine used on the host can be used to mark the donor cornea. Careful measurements should be made. The size is certainly as critical as in penetrating keratoplasty. Too small a donor will be difficult to stretch to fit the gap at the edge, too large a button will tend to bulge and produce astigmatism. Once the button is cut, however, it tends to shrink very slightly, so that when it is first placed on the host bed it may appear slightly too small.

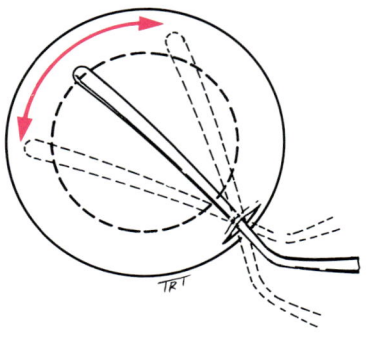

a

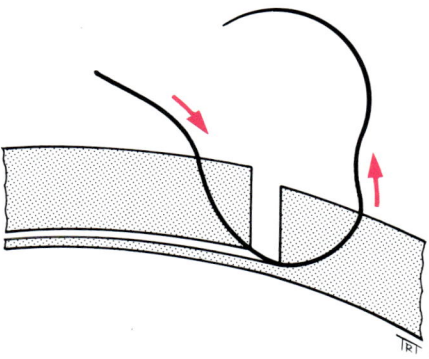

b

Fig. 17.6.

12. The dissection is carried out in an essentially similar fashion. Since the donor is likely to be more oedematous than normal, the surgeon must attempt to make some estimate of the relative disparity between host and donor so that when the donor thins, the cornea should be of normal thickness. The deeper the host dissection has been, the easier this decision will be. Alternatively, the cornea may be dissected at a deep level through a small peripheral pocket using a long curved spatula using long, gentle, sweeping movements. The desired disc of donor tissue may then be cut out (Fig. 17.6).

13. The host bed should be irrigated so that any mucus or blood is removed before the donor is applied.

14. The donor is sutured with 10/0 nylon sutures — either interrupted or continuous. The sutures are passed through the thickness of the button, exiting at the inferior corner and, similarly, are inserted into the deep angle of the host. The correct depth of sutures is thus simple to gauge (Fig. 17.7). The tension should be adjusted to ensure minimal distortion, and the knots buried.

Fig. 17.7.

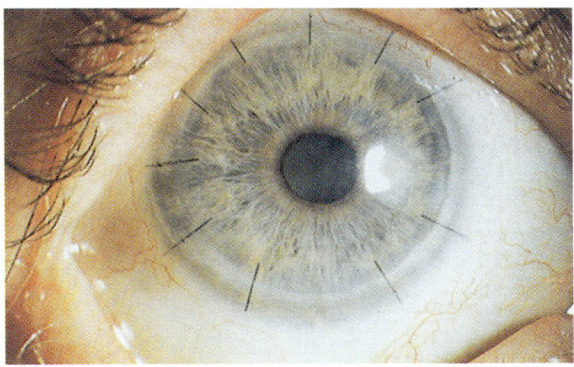

Fig. 17.8.

15. A subconjunctival injection of antibiotic can be given at the end of the procedure. The sutures (Fig. 17.8) can be removed as early as 6 or 12 weeks postoperatively.

Limbal dermoids

The technique of lamellar keratoplasty is ideal for treating (limbal) dermoids. Very rarely, the dermoid involves the full thickness of the eye wall, and is occasionally centrally situated. Most commonly, it is found in the inferotemporal quadrant spanning the limbus. In the rare event of the wound edge being in the optical zone of the cornea, it is wiser to extend the wound beyond so that the optical zone is included in the graft.

1. The conjunctiva should be opened close to the dermoid, and any bleeding controlled.

2. The smallest trephine which will fit around the dermoid is chosen to mark the globe (Fig. 17.9). Sometimes, the dermoid is rather elongated, and tapers off at the scleral end. If this is so, the taper can be gently peeled back a little to accommodate a smaller trephine.

3. The groove is deepened at the corneal edge and the lamellar dissection begun from the most central part of the cornea (close to the dermoid). Usually, the depth needs to be at least two-thirds of the cornea, but the dissection must pass underneath the dermoid (Fig. 17.10). The authors do not recommend 'shaving-off' the dermoid.

4. Once the sclera is reached, there may be a little bleeding at the limbus; this can be controlled with diathermy. The scleral dissection continues at the same depth but, of course, there is no plane of

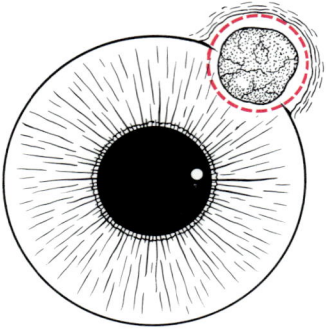

Fig. 17.9.

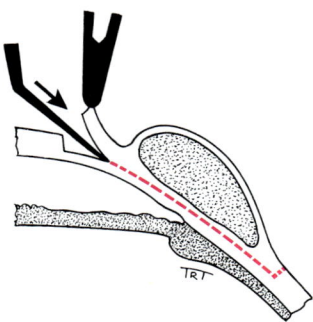

Fig. 17.10.

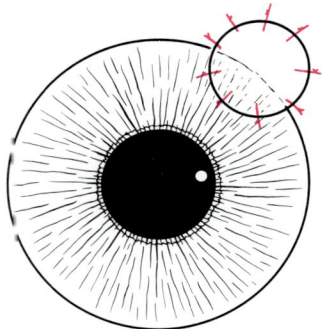

Fig. 17.11.

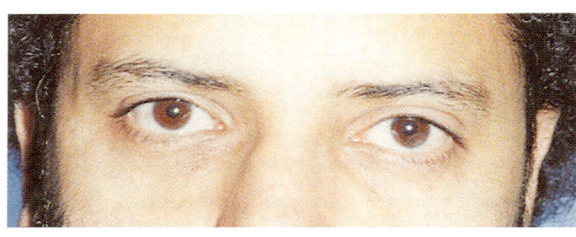

a

Fig. 17.12

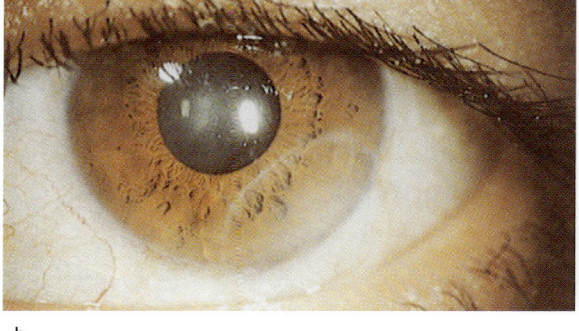

b

dissection. The procedure then resembles the preparation of a scleral flap for trabeculectomy.

5. The donor is prepared as described above. There is no need to attempt matching sclera to sclera. A disc of clear cornea gives an excellent cosmetic result. Interrupted sutures may be easier to remove later (Figs 17.11 and 17.12).

6. The conjunctiva may then be brought up to the edge of the graft, or may form a partial hood and be brought up to the limbus; it appears not to matter which method is used.

COMPLICATIONS

1. If the sutures are not removed at about 3 months, there is a tendency for them to loosen and cause irritation, predisposing to vascularization or infection.

2. Nearly every case of lamellar graft for dermoid shows some minor

degree of interface haemorrhage in the first few days after surgery. This resorbs spontaneously and requires no intervention.

3. Late interface vascularization is uncommon, but should be treated with intense topical steroids should it develop. Its appearance is unsightly but it is otherwise innocent.

18

Surgery for pterygium

Any condition for which there are many different surgical approaches is bound to be controversial, and the greater the number of different operations the less successful an individual procedure is likely to be. The authors will make no attempt to cover all the different permutations that have been employed in the management of this condition. Having been impressed with the results from one particular approach, this will be described.

The presence of a pterygium is not, per se, an indication for removal. Careless removal often results in recurrence which is cosmetically much worse than the original lesion. Tethered globes and a pterygium crossing the axis are uncommon de novo, but not unusual in recurrences.

Where there has been previous surgical interference and the cornea has been unduly thinned, a lamellar graft may be necessary. This can be a 'patch' where the pterygium is not extensive, but may need to include most of the area of the cornea, in some cases extending over the visual axis.

SURGICAL TECHNIQUE

1. A drop of adrenaline 0.1% applied at the beginning of the procedure reduces bleeding.

2. The corneal limits of the pterygium are marked — usually freehand (Fig. 18.1) and the dissection is begun from the most central part of the lesion (Fig. 18.2). The entirety of the leading edge should be included. The minimal depth necessary for complete excision should be chosen. This is probably as important as any step in the operation. Often, the inexperienced surgeon dissects much deeper into the stroma beneath Bowman's layer than is necessary, thereby encouraging recurrence.

3. A virgin pterygium will strip off easily. For a recurrence, a lamellar dissection will be necessary. In any case, the dissection is carried to

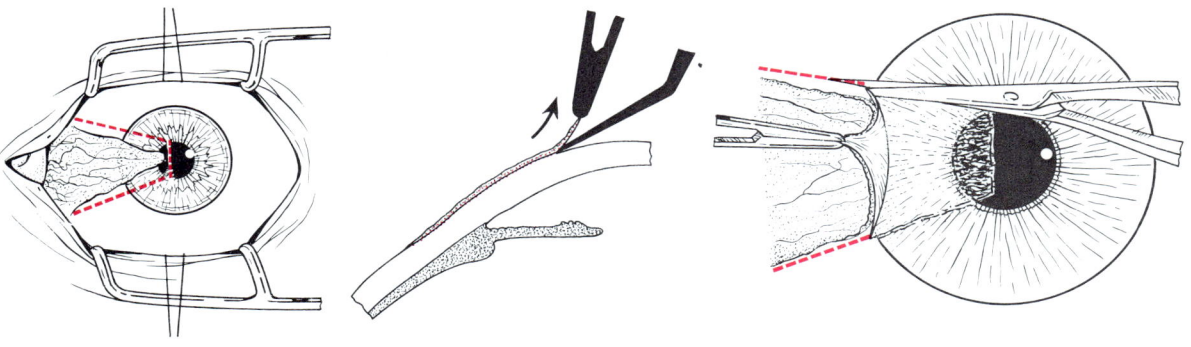

Fig. 18.1.　　　　　Fig. 18.2.　　　　　Fig. 18.3.

the limbus, and once this is reached the lesion lifts very easily from the episcleral tissue.

4. It is impractical, if not impossible, to remove the whole of the lesion as it imperceptibly merges with the conjunctiva of the fornix and plica. The conjunctival portion of the lesion can be excised with scissors (Fig. 18.3). The plica, in particular, should not be disturbed. If this occurs, the scarring and distortion that ensues will produce a very unpleasant cosmetic result, even if there is no recurrence. Similarly, if the dissection is carried too far into the fornices, these will be shallowed and symblepharon may be produced.

5. Bleeding is controlled with diathermy.

6. The pterygium is amputated.

7. If the other eye is healthy, it may be chosen as the site for donor conjunctiva; if not, the upper opposite quadrant of the same eye will suffice. The results appear identical.

8. The conjunctiva is dissected from the underlying Tenon's capsule. Usually 5×8 mm is all that is necessary, but the base of the patch at the limbus should match as nearly as possible the extent of the bare area at the limbus left by the pterygium.

9. The excised patch of conjunctiva is transferred to the bare area, and sutured limbus to limbus with 8/0 virgin silk sutures at each corner.

10. The free conjunctival graft is then stretched out to cover the bare area. It can be helped in this task by reticulating it with tiny cuts with fine-pointed scissors. The resultant net stretches to cover a wide area, and also prevents the build-up of transudate under the graft (Fig. 18.4).

11. The graft and host conjunctival edges are sutured together with 8/0

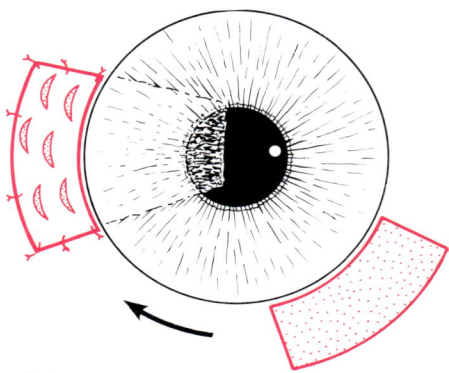

Fig. 18.4.

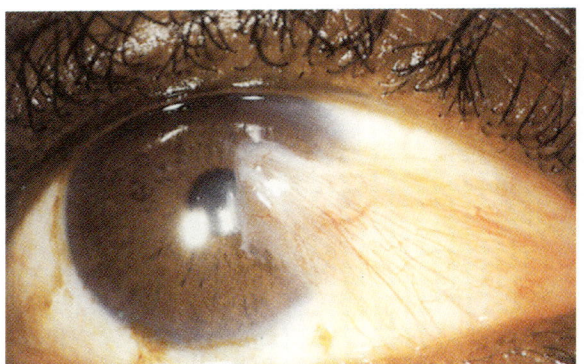

Fig. 18.5.

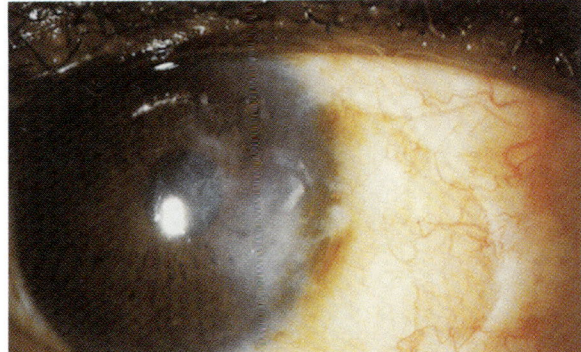

Fig. 18.6.

virgin silk. The donor site re-epithelializes quickly, and the graft rapidly establishes itself, producing a very satisfactory appearance.

At the end of the procedure, antibiotic ointment is instilled and the eye padded for 48 hours. Topical antibiotic and steroid drops are used for about 6 weeks.

Any tendency for invasion of the cornea by blood vessels can be treated with an argon laser. Figures 18.5 and 18.6 show the typical pre- and postoperative appearances.

19

Ocular surface modifying procedures

Conjunctival flap

The conjunctival flap is an excellent procedure for bringing comfort and stability to eyes which are painful from intractable ocular surface disease, and which are blind or have poor visual expectation. Although it may be possible to undo the flap at a later stage, this is usually difficult and unsatisfactory since the limbal stem cells have been largely destroyed, and re-epithelialization will be slow and unhealthy. In general terms, the flap, once formed, *should be intended to be permanent*.

The key to success is to avoid 'buttonholing' (i.e. perforating the conjunctiva as it is dissected) at all costs, and at the same time dissecting the conjunctiva so that only the conjunctiva is split off from Tenon's capsule, which is left undisturbed. The result will also be better if the conjunctiva does not have to be stretched over the cornea.

The conjunctiva will not stick down to the cornea if the corneal epithelium is left in situ. If corneal epithelium is left behind, inclusion cysts may form. The epithelium may be removed at the beginning of the operation, or else left until the conjunctival dissection has been completed.

SURGICAL TECHNIQUE

1. The dissection is started by making two small relieving incisions behind the limbus at 8 and 4 o'clock. Using fine scissors, such as Wescot's spring scissors, the conjunctiva is freed by blunt dissection from Tenon's capsule (Fig. 19.1). The points of the scissors are introduced under the conjunctiva, the blades repeatedly opened and closed, forming a pocket, so that the fine septa can be cut. The procedure is repeated circumferentially around the limbus towards the 12 o'clock position.

2. As the conjunctiva is freed, a peritomy at the limbus can be made, but this should always be the last step in dissecting any segment.

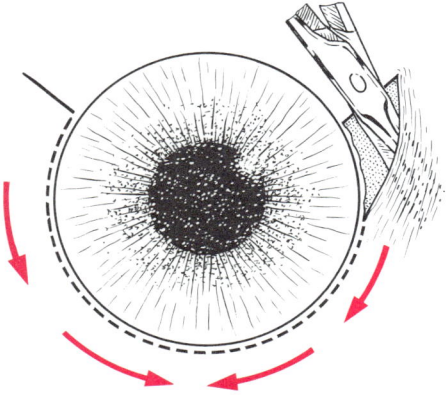

Fig. 19.1.

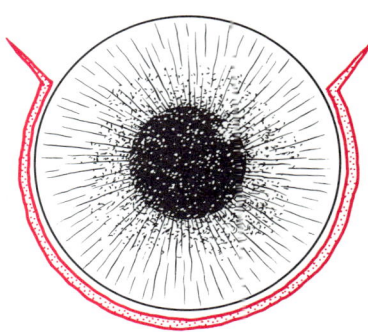

Fig. 19.2.

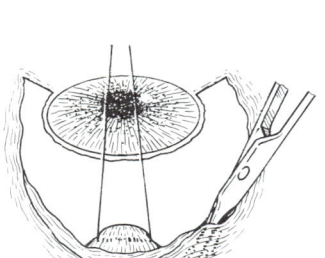

Fig. 19.3.

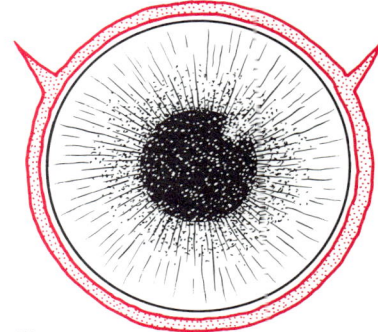

Fig. 19.4.

Eventually, all the superior conjunctiva will be freed (Fig. 19.2) and the dissection needs to be continued into the fornix.

3. At this point, a traction suture may be usefully inserted either in the sclera or in the superior rectus tendon but NOT transfixing the conjunctiva (Fig. 19.3). As the dissection is carried upwards into the fornix, the tissue becomes thicker and it is less easy to confine the dissection to the conjunctiva alone.

4. Eventually, enough conjunctiva will have been freed to cover the cornea completely, i.e. the conjunctiva needs to be brought down right to the inferior limbus. No hard and fast rules can be laid down as to how far the dissection needs to be taken, since the elasticity of the conjunctiva will vary greatly depending on the degree of scarring present. Dissecting too much conjunctiva will produce ptosis. In some cases, this may be unavoidable.

5. Once the superior conjunctiva has been freed, the inferior conjunctiva needs to be dissected in a similar, but less extensive,

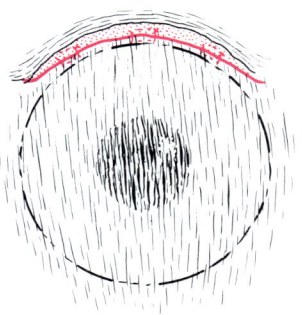

Fig. 19.5.

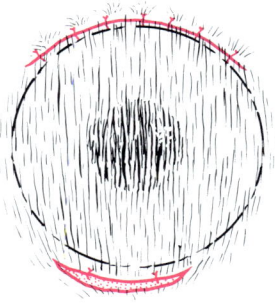

Fig. 19.6.

fashion. It is important not to carry the dissection too deep into the inferior fornix, causing shallowing of the inferior fornix. This will make fitting and wearing of a cosmetic shell more difficult later (Fig. 19.4).

6. The corneal epithelium is now removed. The epithelium can be loosened either with absolute alcohol or cocaine 4% drops. Both these solutions are toxic to the conjunctiva, and there is an advantage in waiting until the conjunctiva has been freed before the application. The cut conjunctival edge can be retracted and protected with cellulose swabs. The solutions are applied to the corneal epithelium with a damp cellulose sponge, and the epithelium debrided with a 'D15', Bard Parker blade. A ring of tissue is likely to remain at the limbus. If left in situ, this is capable of replication and will form inclusion cysts. These limbal remnants can be destroyed by cautery or bipolar diathermy.

7. The superior conjunctival edge is now pulled down to the inferior limbus. Avoid trying to suture the two conjunctival edges together across the cornea, since there is a tendency for them to pull apart, leaving a bare area which may ulcerate. The free superior edge is sutured to the inferior sclera using mattress sutures, which are less likely to pull out under the initial tension. The inferior edge is then brought up and sutured to the superior conjunctival edge with interrupted 8/0 virgin silk sutures which include the sclera. Silk causes minimal irritation, and the slight inflammatory reaction may help to strengthen the suture line (Fig. 19.5).

8. If the flap appears to be under too much tension, a small relieving incision – no more than 10 mm long, or the flap may become ischaemic – can be made at the level of the superior limbus, and the corneal edge of the flap (Fig. 19.6).

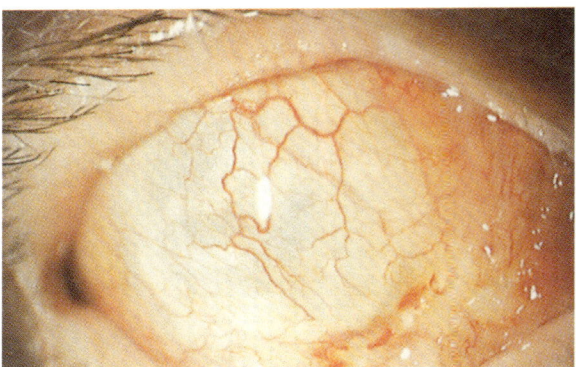

Fig. 19.7.

9. Should any buttonholes have been formed, they should be closed with the finest material available, without creating more buttonholes and with minimal tension. Alternatively, it may be possible to position the flap so that the buttonhole is beyond the limbus. Even if this means additional dissection it is preferable. The flap can then be sutured in the usual fashion behind the buttonhole.

10. At the end of the procedure, antibiotic ointment is instilled, and the eye padded and left undisturbed for 48 hours. This helps to prevent the accumulation of fluid under the flap and aids healing. Topical antibiotic drops can be used for a short time until the wound is healed.

11. A cosmetic shell or soft contact lens can be fitted early, but the flap itself will continue maturing for several months, gradually becoming thinner and less noticeable to the extent that many patients feel that the cosmetic effect is quite acceptable without any shell (Fig. 19.7).

COMPLICATIONS

Providing a buttonhole has not been produced, postoperative problems are rare. A small buttonhole in a flap with no tension may not matter, but usually there is a tendency for the tiny hole to enlarge, undoing the protective effect of the flap. If this becomes a serious problem, a free conjunctival graft from the contralateral eye, or even a free buccal mucous membrane graft, may restore integrity to the ocular surface. Neglected buttonholes may lead to microbial keratitis or corneal perforation.

Inclusion cysts may form after a few months, when there has been inadequate obliteration of the limbal epithelium. When this happens, the cysts can be removed by dissection from the conjunctival side.

Occasionally, a flap covering only a portion of the cornea is required for protection of a peripheral ulcer or corneal melt. These cases require careful assessment, but circumstances may make a flap the only practical solution. The basic technique is similar to that already described, but here the free conjunctival edge will be sutured down to the bare cornea. Central ulcers may require a 'bucket handle' flap. In these cases, where the visual axis has been occluded, the flap can be undone once the underlying condition has been adequately treated. Because the limbus has not been destroyed, epithelial healing should not be impeded. Usually, a keratoplasty will be required after the flap is removed.

In certain difficult situations, e.g. Stevens–Johnson syndrome with perforation, where keratoplasty has been followed by further perforation, regraft can be combined with a conjunctival flap; this may preserve not only the eye but also navigational vision.

Kenyon procedure (free limbal transplant from the contralateral eye or stem cell graft)

In cases where there is extensive unilateral ocular damage, e.g. following an alkali burn where the limbus has been destroyed, re-epithelialization of the cornea takes place slowly, with conjunctivally derived cells supplanting the normal corneal epithelium. Such epithelium is irregular and often heavily vascularized – in effect a pannus extending over the whole cornea. These eyes are very difficult to rehabilitate visually as, until recently, penetrating keratoplasty had an appallingly bad outcome.

SURGICAL TECHNIQUE

Kenyon developed the technique of Thoft (epithelioplasty) to transplant cells from a contralateral healthy limbus. It is now our routine to ascertain that the donor eye is healthy by first performing impression cytology on the donor taking specimens from the bulbar conjunctiva close to the limbus at 12, 3, 6 and 9 o'clock positions.

1. A superficial keratectomy first prepares the host eye in a similar fashion to removing the epithelium for a conjunctival flap. Usually, the pannus strips easily from the underlying stroma. The dissection should be carried back beyond the original limbus.

2. At the 12 and 6 o'clock positions, a circumferential and slightly deeper keratectomy needs to be done through about two clock hours and about 3 mm wide, to prepare a bed for the transplant.

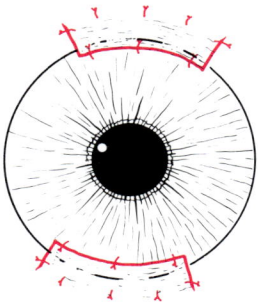

Fig. 19.8.

3. From the donor eye, a similarly shaped piece of tissue needs to be carefully excised, using scissors to free the conjunctival edge, a blade to begin the dissection in the sclera and cornea, and a lamellar dissector such as a Paufique knife. The dissection does not have to be very deep, only deep enough to include the base of the epithelium at the limbus. Taking a few lamellae of cornea and sclera may help to support the tissue, making it manageable and ensuring that the dissection is deep enough.

4. The donor tissue is secured in place with 10/0 or 11/0 nylon interrupted sutures (Fig. 19.8).

Antibiotic ointment is instilled and the eyes padded. The receiving eye should be kept covered for 48 hours, but the patch can be removed from the donating eye the next day and antibiotic drops and weak steroid drops instilled until re-epithelialization has taken place. The donating eye may be more comfortable patched for a few days and, if re-epithelialization is slow, a bandage contact lens (possibly silicone) can be applied. Antibiotic and steroids are instilled until full healing has taken place.

If penetrating keratoplasty is to be attempted, it should be delayed for at least 6 months, and preferably for a year, to allow stabilization. The ocular surface will continue to show maturation for several years.

Limbal transplant – allograft

In circumstances where the contralateral eye is not found to be healthy, either by slitlamp examination or by impression cytology, an allograft must be used as a donor for the stem cells. Although it may be possible to use a stored corneoscleral disc as a donor, the authors have preferred a whole, fresh donor eye as donor. The procedure is technically very similar to that described above but certain variations are possible.

1. If only two single clock hour sections are to be used (as above) then it is important to identify accurately the 12 and 6 o'clock positions where the stem cells are densest. This can be done on an enucleated eye by inspection of the rectus muscle insertions. This technique then follows an identical course to that described above. The donor eye is held in a Croydon eye stand (Pierse–Steele).

2. Since a whole donor eye is being used there is no need to restrict the donor site to just two (separate) clock hours. A ring of donor tissue may be excised in a similar manner. The host site obviously needs to be prepared to match.

3. Alternatively, a larger superficial lamellar graft may be performed. On the whole although technically easier, it is probably not so desirable as there may be difficulties with vascularization and even melting of the donor stroma.

In any case, immune suppression of the host will be necessary. The authors recommend the use of systemic cyclosporin A.

This procedure is contraindicated in cases of significant ocular surface keratinization because keratinization will affect the grafted tissue, resulting in surface opacification.

APPLICATION OF CYANOACRYLATE GLUE

At present, cyanoacrylate glue – n-butyl, isocyanoacrylate (Histacryl™) is not licensed in the United Kingdom for ophthalmic use, and can only be used on a 'named patient' basis. It is, nevertheless, such a useful technique that the authors feel it must be included in this volume.

The main indication for the use of glue is a small perforation in the cornea, not exceeding 1 mm in diameter (Fig. 19.9a, b).

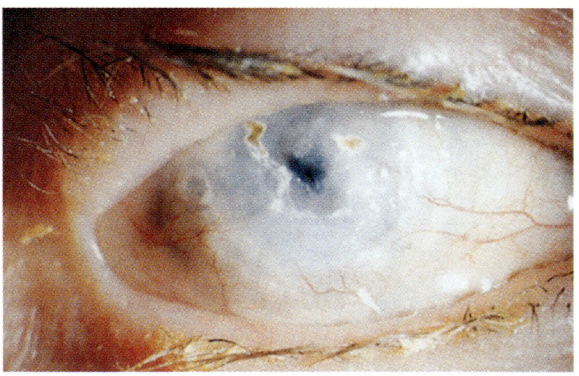

a

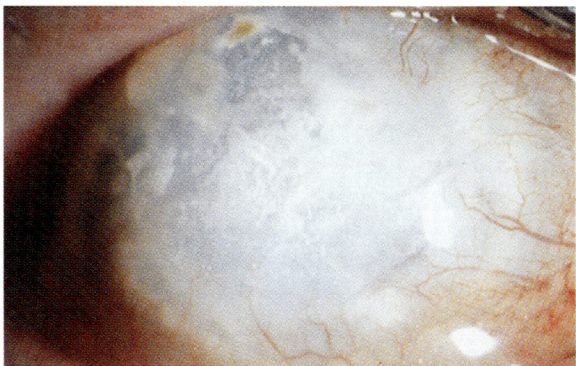

b

Fig. 19.9.

Infection is not an absolute contraindication but, in the authors' experience, perforation in microbial keratitis will ultimately require an emergency graft. Glue may, however, be a useful temporizing measure where a suitable donor is not available.

SURGICAL TECHNIQUE

1. Glue does not stick well to epithelium and, if necessary, a small area of epithelium around the perforation site should be removed.

2. The perforation site must not continue leaking while the glue is being applied. This can be quite difficult to achieve. The aqueous can be absorbed on to a cellulose sponge, but if this fails, a small air bubble or blob of healon can be injected into the anterior chamber through the perforation, with a Rycroft cannula.

3. The glue should be drawn up into a 2-ml syringe and then applied one drop at a time on to the perforation site. It may be easier to drop the glue on to the cornea from the tip of an iris repositor, rather than directly from the syringe. Each drop should have dried (polymerized) before the next is applied. As the glue dries, it becomes a pale opalescent lilac colour and the surface wrinkles (Fig. 19.9b). Several drops may be required to seal the perforation effectively. Patience is required to wait until each drop dries.

4. If the anterior chamber has been lost, it should be restored, once the perforation is secure, through a separate paracentesis site. This allows the watertightness to be checked but, more importantly, it prevents the development of aqueous misdirection syndrome and may help to limit chronic angle closure.

5. At the end of the procedure, a bandage contact lens must be fitted for comfort to the patient. Where the eye is dry, a silicone lens should be used.

The glue permits the normal reparative process to continue and in due course, after a few days to a few weeks, will loosen and fall out. Hopefully it will leave an intact cornea, but if there is still a leak it can be replaced.

BOTULINUM TOXIN PROTECTIVE PTOSIS

A chemically medicated ptosis can cover an ulcer and provide protection to the ulcer, speeding healing with ultimately full recovery of the lid function.

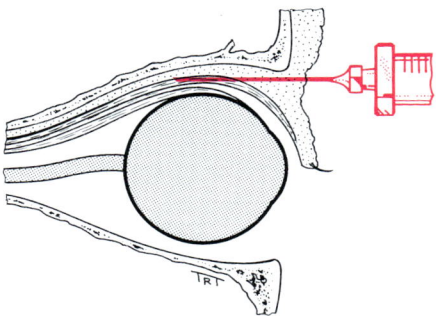

Fig. 19.10.

In the UK, botulinum toxin A (the active agent) has recently been licensed for therapeutic use.

Occasionally, corneal ulcers (which are sterile) are slow to heal for a variety of reasons. Traditionally employed means to aid healing have included lid patching, bandage contact lenses, and tarsorraphy; none of these methods are entirely satisfactory. Tarsorraphy, in particular, carries the risk of permanent damage to the lid margin, which may further prejudice the vulnerable ocular surface.

The toxin injection can also be used prophylactically in cases of acoustic neuroma undergoing neurosurgery, or in Bell's palsy. The toxin is available freeze-dried, and must be reconstituted prior to use. The usual dose of toxin is 62.5 pg in 0.1 ml, but the dose is not crucial and may safely be doubled without risk. No anaesthetic is necessary.

A standard 25 mm, 25 gauge needle is required. The central part of the orbital rim is palpated and, with the patient looking down, the needle is passed straight back along the roof of the orbit to its full length and the toxin injected (Fig. 19.10). The injection may be repeated if necessary. Until the lid drops in about 2 or 3 days, the full ancillary supportive measures must be continued.

Photorefractive therapeutic keratectomy (PTK)

The development of the excimer laser which is able to be applied to a corneal surface is a tool of immense refinement. Each laser pulse can be expected to remove tissue at a depth of no more than 0.2 of a micron. This facility has been found to be of great value, not only in the refractive world (dealt with in later chapters), but also for corneal surface modification. The list of conditions which can be helped by this procedure is extensive, but includes superficial corneal scarring, superficial opacities related to stromal dystrophies, epithelial instability related to anterior limiting membrane dystrophies, the flattening of small proud nebulae interfering with contact lens wear (particularly in patients with keratoconus), and band shaped keratopathy.

The laser is applied to the surface of the cornea after previous removal of the overlying epithelium, and the amount of laser application varies considerably depending upon the condition being treated. For those patients requiring no more than five to ten pulses of laser, e.g. recurrent erosions, there is no significant effect on the patient's refractive error. For patients, however, requiring somewhat deeper surface modification, e.g. corneal dystrophy or band shaped keratopathy, there is a tendency for the procedure to be followed by some degree of hypermetropia. Apart from the very early postoperative period, which is necessarily uncomfortable until the epithelium has re-healed, there are no significant complications. It should be noted that vascularized superficial disorders are not satisfactory for treatment by this modality as the laser treatment will cause bleeding which cannot be easily controlled and which interferes with the application of the laser.

Section D
Refractive surgery

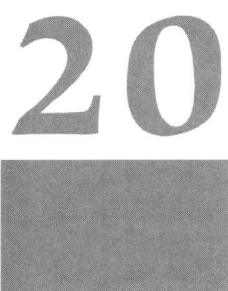

Correction of post-graft astigmatism

The success of corneal grafting depends not only upon the maintenance of a clear and healthy graft, but also on the ability of the patient to enjoy good vision through it. A corneal graft's refractive state becomes reasonably stable 3 months after surgery. At this time, glasses or contact lenses may be prescribed if the patient achieves good vision with a wearable refractive correction. Sometimes it is not possible to prescribe, because of a high degree of regular astigmatism.

ASSESSMENT

The refractive error should be assessed by retinoscopy and subjective refraction, usefully verified by keratometry and videokeratoscopy – see Chapter 2.

Indications for surgery

EARLY POSTOPERATIVE PERIOD

When a patient is dependent on good vision through the corneal graft as soon as possible after surgery, perhaps because of serious ocular disorder in the other eye, it is necessary to modify the shape of the corneal graft without interfering with the sutures already in place. This problem should be treated by the addition of further interrupted 10/0 nylon sutures placed in the axis of the flat meridian (Fig. 20.1). These sutures should be turned so that the knot enters the suture track in the corneal stroma. This minor operation requires full sterile conditions, but can be done quite satisfactorily using topical (preservative-free) anaesthesia only. The alteration of the shape of the graft as a result of the insertion of extra sutures may be monitored perioperatively by the use of a simple qualitative surgical keratometer, such as the reflection of a circular object placed between the microscope and the centre of the surface of the graft. The addition of extra sutures should be stopped

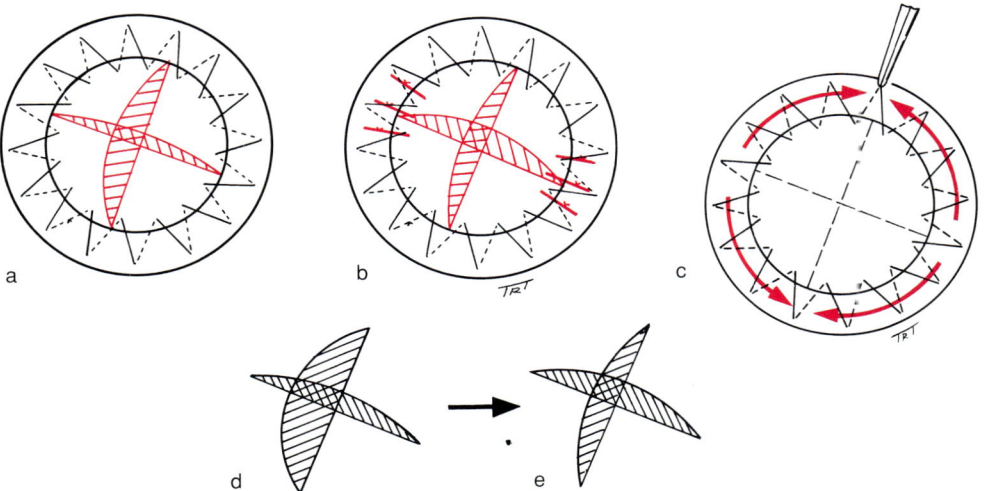

Fig. 20.1.

when the undesired oval reflection has been converted to circular. In this case it is undesirable to overcorrect the refractive error, as the patient needs to achieve good vision immediately.

It is advisable, following such a minor disturbance of the corneal graft, to increase the dosage of local steroid and antibiotic medication for 2 or 3 weeks postoperatively, to lessen the chance of graft rejection.

An alternative technique for managing significant early astigmatism developing within the first 6 postoperative weeks is to manipulate the tension of the running suture. This may be done at the slitlamp, using topical anaesthesia. It requires great care in handling the suture. Plain forceps with smooth edges, or a fine-tipped, smooth-edged needle-holder are used. The suture is held and gently pulled in its own line. The steep axis must be flattened by pulling the suture towards it, i.e. starting at each end of the flat axis of the graft (Fig. 20.1).

LATE POSTOPERATIVE PERIOD

Removal of graft suture(s)

If at the 12-month postoperative stage a patient enjoys good vision through the corneal graft with the graft suture in situ, there is no need to remove it. If, however, a patient is prevented from using the corneal graft at this stage because of a refractive error which includes a significant amount of astigmatism, the graft suture, if it is continuous, should be removed.

If, on the other hand, the graft has been performed using interrupted sutures, the astigmatism may be reduced at any time from the sixth to

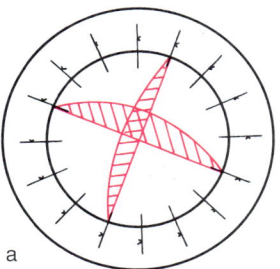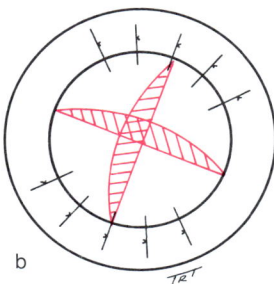

Fig. 20.2.

eighth postoperative month by the selective removal of sutures one at a time from the axis of the steepest curvature. Once the refractive error can be controlled in this manner, the removal of sutures should be discontinued. Remember that the object of the exercise is not to eliminate astigmatism, but to reduce the refractive error to one which can be corrected by either a spectacle or contact lens (Fig. 20.2).

Reassessment

If removal of the graft sutures fails to correct the problem of post-graft astigmatism, further surgery will be required. The graft wound is carefully inspected along its circumference for areas of uneven healing and, in particular, for signs of stretching of the wound in the axis of the flat meridian. Such stretching may occur because of uneven graft suture tensions, premature removal of graft sutures, an area of thin peripheral stroma, or an area of host stromal vascularization where the sutures will frequently loosen early.

  If wound weakness is located aligned with the flat axis, this is almost certainly the cause of the astigmatic problem and it is therefore to this area that the treatment is best directed.

Surgical technique

Under sterile conditions and local topical anaesthesia, the wound in the stretched area is re-deepened with a diamond knife. It is best to avoid opening the anterior chamber if possible. The re-opening of the wound should extend for between 30 and 60° of the circumference, depending upon the degree of astigmatism and the length of weak wound identified. The re-opened wound should then be closed using 4–8 interrupted sutures of 9/0 nylon. The sutures should be placed relatively close together to allow for flexibility at a later stage. The degree of correction should be monitored perioperatively by the use of a qualitative keratometer, as described above. The original astigmatic error will be seen as an oval reflection rather than a circular one and the

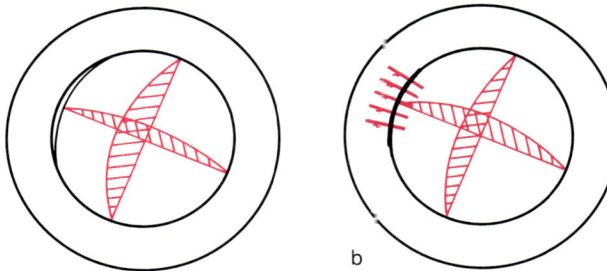

Fig. 20.3.

a   b

long axis of the oval will correspond to the flat axis of the cornea. As the sutures are inserted, so the shape of the oval reflection will alter; but in this case a deliberate attempt must be made to overcorrect the refractive error so that the refractive sutures will produce a steep axis in their own meridian. These sutures are now left in situ for at least three months. The patient needs to be warned that this procedure takes some time to produce its beneficial refractive result (Fig. 20.3).

At the conclusion of the procedure, the patient should be treated for 2–3 weeks with an increased level of both topical steroid and antibiotic. After 3 months, if the overcorrection has been maintained, the refractive sutures may be removed one at a time; the suture chosen is always the one closest to the axis of the now steep meridian. One suture per month only should be removed. When the refractive error has been reduced to a degree where it can be corrected either by a spectacle or contact lens, the process of suture removal should be stopped and the remaining sutures left in place indefinitely. The advantage of 9/0 nylon is that it is less liable to biodegradation and able to remain in place for several years.

If, after removal of the original graft suture, careful inspection of the wound circumference fails to locate an area of wound stretching, other techniques for reducing the astigmatism must be employed.

Relieving incisions (Arcuate Keratotomy)
Under sterile conditions and with topical local anaesthesia only, one or two curved incisions are made either in the graft wound or into the stroma immediately central to the graft wound. These incisions are approximately 60° in length and are placed to be centred on the axis of steepest curvature. These relaxing incisions should flatten the steep axis. The effect of the incision may be observed perioperatively by the use of a simple qualitative keratometer, the same reflected circular object as described above. The long axis of the oval reflection will correspond to the flat axis, and if the relieving incisions are to be effective, a change in

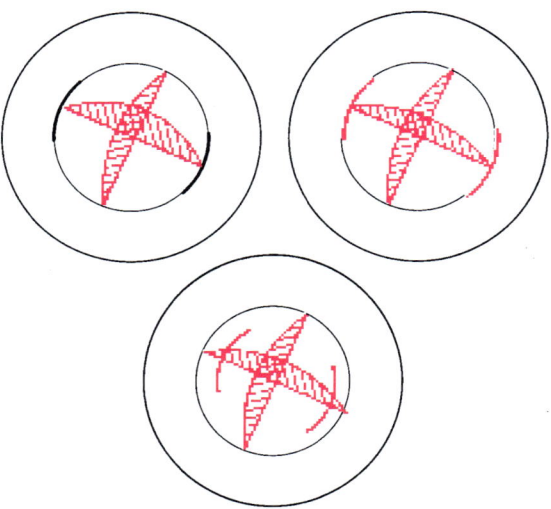

Fig. 20.4.

the shape of the cornea will be observable immediately. The incisions are made to a depth just short of perforating the anterior chamber. When the incisions have been correctly placed and are effective, the edges of the incisions will gape very slightly immediately after the incision has been made. This sign will almost certainly be associated with a demonstrable alteration of the corneal curvature. Under these circumstances no further surgery is required, and the patients should be treated with steroid and antibiotic drops for at least 3 weeks following the procedure. The refractive error will probably stabilize within 1 week (Fig. 20.4).

Relieving incisions with reinforcing sutures

When the procedure above fails to produce an alteration of corneal curvature, or where the alteration of shape is unlikely to be sufficient for corrective purposes, the relieving incisions should be augmented by the insertion of two reinforcing sutures, one placed on each side of the graft in the axis of the greatest flattening. These sutures should be of 9/0 nylon and must be inserted with sufficient tension to produce a definite overcorrection of the preoperative refractive error. When in place, the tension from the reinforcing sutures will be seen to produce a parting of the surface lips of the relieving incisions previously made. Following this procedure, the patient should be treated for 3 weeks with an increased level of local steroid and antibiotic drops. The reinforcing sutures should be left in situ for 6 weeks, after which time they may be removed one at a time with an intervening interval of not less than 1 month. If after removal of one of the sutures the patient's refractive

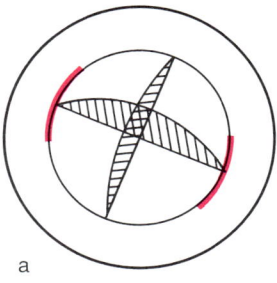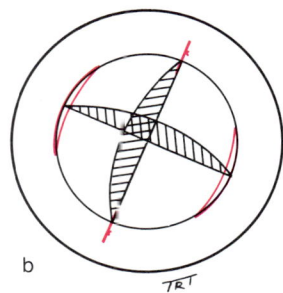

Fig. 20.5.

error is seen to have been sufficiently corrected, the other suture should be left in place indefinitely (Fig. 20.5).

Refractive resuturing

Refractive resuturing is indicated when relieving incisions have failed to help sufficiently. This process is exactly the same as for cases where an area of graft wound weakness has been located. An area of wound for re-opening and resuturing is chosen, centred on the flat axis. These refractive sutures will steepen the flat axis, and the sutures must be introduced to produce a definite over-correction of the preoperative refractive error. Occasionally, it may be necessary to have two areas of refractive resuturing placed at each end of the flat axis. This is for the correction of very high degrees of post-graft astigmatism (Fig. 20.6).

The treatment of the post-graft astigmatism is completed when it is possible to prescribe a correcting and wearable spectacle or contact lens.

Some authorities have advocated the use of Ruiz type procedures for the management of post-graft astigmatism. The authors do not recommend these techniques as they involve surgery into the host peripheral cornea outside the graft wound. In the event of the graft subsequently failing and requiring replacement, such peripheral refractive surgery could cause problems.

Excimer laser correction

For patients whose astigmatism is associated with residual myopia there is a temptation to use the excimer laser as a correcting modality. The benefits in theory are the simultaneous elimination of both the myopic and the astigmatic elements. The problems are that accurate elimination of high astigmatic errors is difficult to achieve and there is a risk of increased subepithelial haze formation in the grafted tissue across the visual axis. The technique is employed occasionally. More recently,

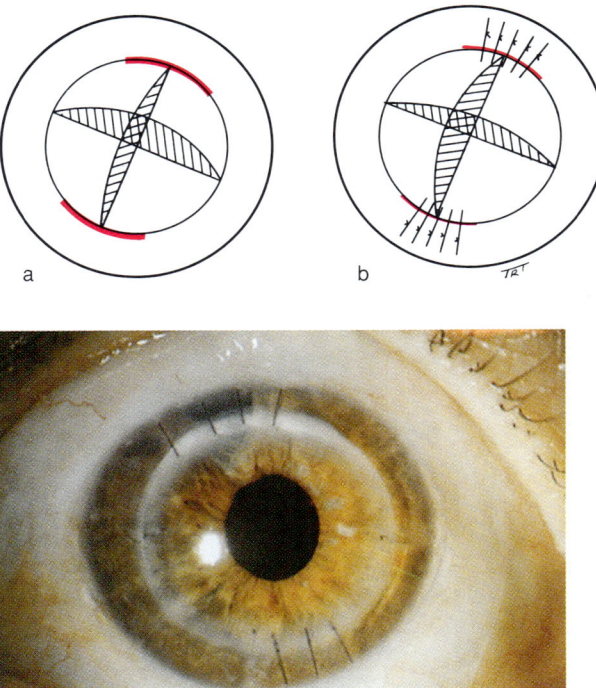

Fig. 20.6.

surface PRK has been replaced by a LASIK procedure in order to achieve the same benefit. The benefit of these highly experimental techniques remain to be proven.

SUMMARY

Surgeons, therefore, have a choice of techniques available to them for handling this all too common complication. In the absence of severe wound weakness, the authors favour relieving incisions within the graft substance, usually using a diameter of separation of 6 mm, arc lengths of $60°$ and an incision depth of 0.6 mm. This simple technique will correct most cases.

21

Radial keratotomy

INDICATIONS

Radial keratotomy is a procedure for removing low degrees of myopia of between 1 and 6 dioptres. The procedure may also be used for myopes of more than 6 dioptres, but these patients can expect a partial correction only. With more than 12 dioptres of myopia, it is unlikely that the degree of correction achieved will be enough to be of value to the patient. For those who have an associated astigmatic error, a preoperative astigmatism of greater than 2 dioptres much reduces the chance of achieving good uncorrected visual acuity. Such patients are probably best discouraged from undergoing radial keratotomy. Patients under the age of 20 should not have refractive surgery because of the likelihood of their developing further myopia up to the age of 21 or 22. Few patients over the age of 55 present for refractive surgery for myopia. Those that do often act in the belief that the surgery will improve their corrected visual acuity. These patients also should be actively discouraged.

PATIENT ASSESSMENT

Patients wishing to undergo radial keratotomy, and who meet the indications, need to be assessed for previous or current ocular disorder other than the myopia. In most cases, associated eye disease affecting either the anterior or posterior segment of the eye will be a contra-indication for radial keratotomy. However, this should not include those patients who have experienced difficulties with contact lens wear due to loss of tolerance. In particular, patients should not be considered for radial keratotomy if they show the slightest evidence of lens changes likely to lead to the development of cataract. For these patients, management of the myopia can be undertaken simultaneously with the eventual cataract surgery, by the selection of an appropriate intraocular lens.

Radial keratotomy patients should understand that this procedure, like many other forms of refractive surgery, is best regarded as experimental. No one is yet able to accurately predict the long-term outcome of this procedure. Patients require a careful explanation of the procedure, emphasizing the known disadvantages resulting from the surgery — weakening of the corneal structure together with the lowering of resistance to corneal infection. It is now clear that this latter problem may extend for many years postoperatively. Finally, patients should be instructed that no guarantee can be provided by the surgeon that the procedure will result in the desired degree of refractive change.

PREOPERATIVE MEASUREMENTS

Refraction
The surgeon requires an accurate preoperative refraction, and this is best done at a time when the patient has been without a contact lens for not less than 2 days.

Pachometry
Measurements of corneal thickness are best undertaken preoperatively, and measurements should be made both centrally and at four to eight points in the mid-corneal periphery. Corneal thickness can be surprisingly variable, and this measurement should also be undertaken at a time when the patient has been without contact lenses not less than 2 days. Perioperative pachometry, in the author's experience, has no added value for the procedure and, in fact, has a number of technical disadvantages.

Intraocular pressure
It is helpful to know whether a patient's intraocular pressure is on the high or low side of normal. Patients with an intraocular pressure of between 15 and 21 mmHg tend to have a greater response to surgery than those at the lower end of the pressure scale.

DETERMINATION OF SURGERY REQUIRED

The incisions of radial keratotomy lead to the steepening of the peripheral corneal curvature and an associated flattening of the central corneal curvature. It is, of course, this flattening that corrects the myopia. There are three surgical variables which need to be determined before the operation commences:

1. The number of incisions

Most surgeons now employ either four or eight radially placed incisions. For patients with preoperative myopia of less than 3 dioptres, four incisions will frequently suffice. For patients with 3 dioptres of myopia or more, eight incisions will usually be required. It is now rare for surgeons to employ 16 incisions, as were originally described.

2. Size of central clear zone

The central clear zone may vary in size from 5 to 3 mm. There are, therefore, five choices of central spared area, assuming intervening steps of not less than 0.5 mm.

3. Depth of incisions

Radial keratotomy is only successful when the incisions are made as deep as possible. In most cases, therefore, the surgeon's knife with its micrometer control may be set at a depth equal to 115% of the measured central corneal thickness. This setting should, of course, be checked with the measurements made of peripheral corneal thickness, and may be modified up or down according to any obvious disparity.

Two other factors are also taken into consideration at this stage:

4. The patient's age
5. The patient's sex

HOW MUCH SURGERY TO DO?

Surgeons may have recourse to a wide variety of nomograms to assist with the determination of how much surgery should be sufficient for an individual patient. The author, however, has for the last 6 years successfully used a formula of great simplicity. For an average patient (male, aged 27), eight incisions with a central clear zone of 3.5 mm will correct 3.5 dioptres of myopia. Patients with more than 3.5 dioptres of myopia will therefore require eight incisions and a 3-mm clear zone, while patients with less than 3.5 dioptres of myopia may have a central clear zone of 4 mm or even 4.5–5.0 mm. It is now known that female patients tend to need relatively more surgery than males of the same age, and that younger patients require relatively more surgery for the same degree of myopia than older patients. At the same time, for patients who are deemed to require four incisions only, the central spared area will need to be 0.5 mm smaller than if they were undergoing eight incisions. This therefore means that patients having four incisions only will never have a central clear zone of greater than 4.5 mm, except perhaps in a male in the older age group of 40–55 years.

PREOPERATIVE MEDICATION

For 1 hour before surgery the patient should have three instillations of pilocarpine 4% drops to achieve a tight miosis.

SURGICAL TECHNIQUE

1. Anaesthesia
Radial keratotomy may be undertaken using either a general or a local anaesthetic. The safety of the procedure is considerably increased if the patient is deprived of all power of voluntary eye movement. The author's preference is for a general anaesthetic, though it is realized that this is frequently impractical for many surgeons.

2. Skin preparation and draping
This operation should always be carried out with proper surgical facilities to eliminate the risks of misadventure and to reduce, as much as possible, the risk of surgical infection. The skin of the eyelids and surrounding face should be prepared using an iodine- or chlorhexidine-based solution. It is not necessary for the eyelashes to be trimmed. After skin preparation, the patient is draped in the normal manner for an ocular procedure, including the application of an occluding adhesive plastic surgical drape, best applied with the eye open. An incision is then made in the drape to open the interpalpebral aperture so that, with small cuts at each end, the plastic drape may be tucked underneath the lid margin to preclude the lashes of both lids from the surgical field.

3. Speculum
The author prefers a light wire speculum of the Pierse or Barraquer variety. Providing the open speculum allows a complete view of the cornea, it should not be necessary to insert rectus sutures.

4. Determination and marking of the visual axis
The surgeon should ensure that he has a direct and vertical view of the cornea through the surgical microscope. The centre of the miosed pupil is an excellent guide to the position of the visual axis, and is, in fact more accurate than determination of the visual axis by asking the patient to look directly into a co-axial light source. Using a blunt

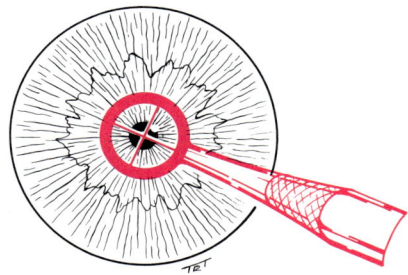

Fig. 21.1.

pointed instrument, a small mark may be made upon the epithelium at this point.

5. Marking the limits of the clear zone

Using a marking circle of the appropriate diameter, the limits of the central clear zone may be marked upon the dry corneal epithelium (Fig. 21.1). Usually, these markers have central crosswires which can be lined up on the mark at the centre of the pupil, as above. Firm pressure on the corneal epithelium will leave a circular depression which will be visible for the duration of the surgical procedure, providing the cornea is kept dry. Before proceeding further, it is wise to measure, with a pair of callipers, the size of the circular mark achieved and check this against a steel rule. Circles made in this way are frequently larger than expected, and failure to detect this enlargement may lead to a disappointing surgical result.

6. Setting the knife

The desired depth is set using the micrometer gauge in the handle of the knife. The diamond blade should now be advanced between the shoulders, and the tip of the diamond should be inspected to ensure that there has been no damage which could limit the depth of cut. The degree to which the diamond tip extends below the shoulders can be verified in a separate gauge if the surgeon does not trust his micrometer. Most of these gauges, however, are so plagued by errors of parallax that they are less accurate than the knife's micrometer.

7. Performing the radial incisions

Depending upon the shape of the diamond blade available to the surgeon, the incisions may be made either from the central clear zone limit to the periphery or vice-versa. Whichever way is chosen, it is essential to remember that the depth of incision adjacent to the central spared area must be to the full depth of the extended blade.

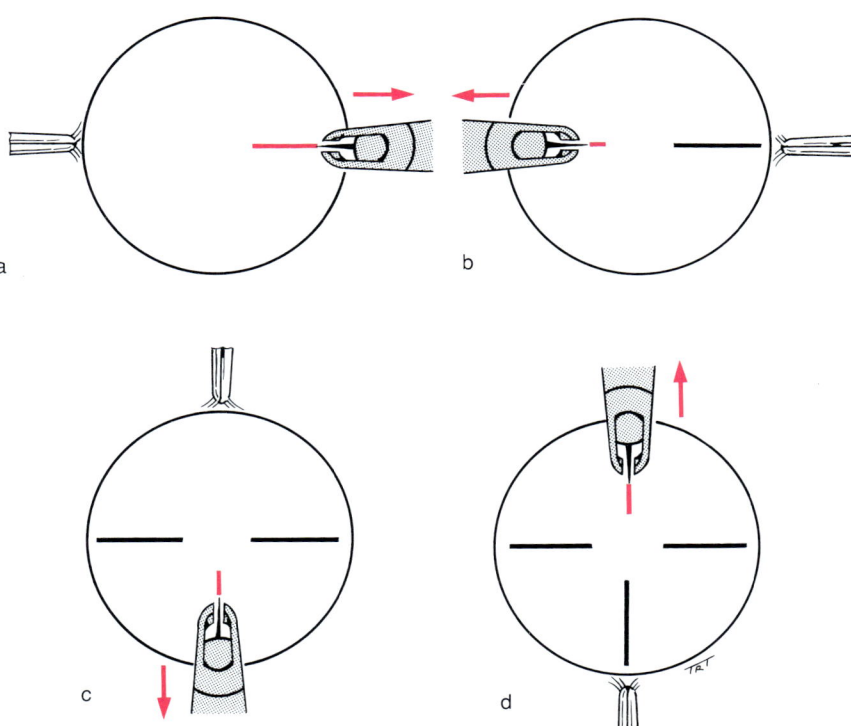

Fig. 21.2.

1. With a pair of toothed collibri forceps, grasp the eye firmly at the limbus at the 3 o'clock position, using the left hand. With the diamond knife in the right hand, an incision is made at the 9 o'clock meridian. The author prefers making the incisions from the centre to the periphery. Ensure that the knife at all times is moving in a straight line in line with the fixing forceps. At the periphery, the incision must end before reaching the surgical limbus, so that a small clear area of uncut cornea remains. After inserting the knife at the central clear zone edge, ensure that the knife is inserted to the full depth of the blade and that the shoulders are resting on the surface of the cornea before moving the knife towards the periphery (Fig. 21.2a).

2. With the fixation forceps in the right hand, and the diamond knife in the left, the eye is grasped at the 9 o'clock limbus adjacent to the end of the incision just made. The knife now makes a matching incision in the 3 o'clock meridian, ensuring that the straight line is accurately aligned with the incision opposite (Fig. 21.2b).

3. With the forceps in the left hand, grasp the limbus at the 6 o'clock position and, with the knife in the right hand, make an incision as

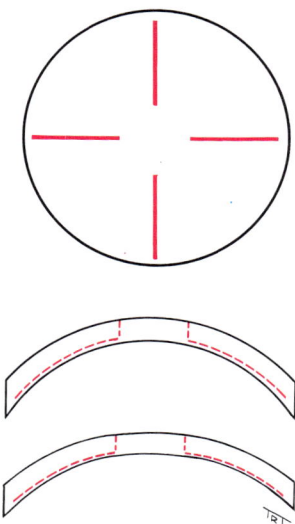

Fig. 21.3.

before in the 12 o'clock meridian. Remember that each incision should stop before reaching the surgical limbus (Fig. 21.2c).

4. Grasp the limbus at 12 o'clock with the forceps, and make an incision in the 6 o'clock meridian (Figs 21.2d and 21.3).

None of these incisions should result in any bleeding. Patients who have been wearing contact lenses for many years before undergoing surgery may have some exaggeration of the limbal vasculature encroaching on to the normal cornea, and in these cases it is difficult to avoid cutting some of these vessels, particularly at the 12 o'clock meridian. For patients requiring eight incisions, four further incisions are made, accurately spaced half-way between the four incisions now established. If a surgeon has difficulty judging accurately the placement of these incisions, or finds it difficult to maintain a straight line, an indenter may be purchased which will impress upon the dry cornea a pattern of eight lines which the surgeon may then follow. It is, however, difficult during the procedure to see ahead of the moving blade, because the knife's shoulders tend to obscure the view. For patients who have retained some eye movement during the operation, due to inadequate anaesthesia, a pair of forceps which fixes the limbus at opposite poles of a meridian may be used. In this case, the forceps grasping the limbus at the 12 and 6 o'clock positions is used to steady fixation while making the incisions in the 3 and 9 o'clock meridians, and so on. In the author's experience, however, these forceps have nothing to offer when a patient is adequately anaesthetised, and the design of the forceps tends to tear the limbus tissues more than a pair of simple toothed collibri forceps.

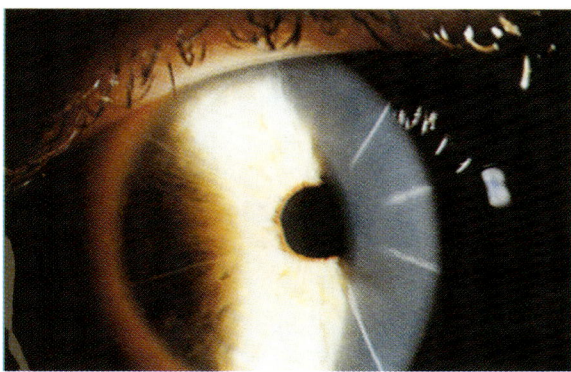

Fig. 21.4.

It will be found that, whichever forceps are used, as the operation proceeds, in order to achieve an adequate depth, the diamond knife will produce corneal indentation. This must be counteracted by applying some pressure to the eye with the fixation forceps, thereby raising the intraocular pressure and limiting the indentation by the knife. A significant degree of indentation will, of course, result in incisions of inadequate depth.

8. Irrigation
Using a syringe filled with normal saline, and a wide-bore Southampton cannula, the incisions are irrigated from the centre towards the periphery to wash out any epithelial debris which may have been carried into the depth of the wound by the knife blade.

9. Drops and dressing
Following the irrigation, drops of a suitable antibiotic, such as chloramphenicol, are instilled into the eye, which is then padded over a melanine pad or tulle gras. The eye should be left padded overnight (Fig. 21.4).

PERIOPERATIVE COMPLICATIONS

Corneal perforation
Despite the care taken (as discussed above) to avoid this problem, corneal perforation will occasionally occur in areas of unexpected thinness. Most commonly, this occurs in the lower temporal quadrant quite close to the point at which the incision is commenced (i.e. the central end of the incision). Providing the cornea and the diamond knife are kept dry at all times throughout the procedure, a spot perforation will be recognized as soon as it occurs. The knife is immediately

withdrawn, and this usually results in no further leakage of aqueous from the anterior chamber. Firstly, the length of the cutting blade on the diamond knife is reduced by 0.02 mm. Secondly, the surgeon proceeds to complete all remaining incisions, leaving the incision with the spot perforation until last. Thirdly, the incision with the spot perforation is completed; although this may result in slight leakage of aqueous due to corneal deformation, the perforation should not be enlarged. It is extremely rare for a spot perforation to be followed by leakage of aqueous once the knife has been withdrawn. However, in the event of persistent leakage, the incision needs to be closed with a single 10/0 suture placed across the incision at the point of the perforation; the knot of the suture is rotated into the corneal stroma, and the suture should be removed 2 or 3 days later without mishap.

Haemorrhage from limbal vessels

Care must be taken to leave a small clear zone between the peripheral extremity of each incision and the surgical limbus. Despite this precaution, haemorrhage from limbal vessels will occasionally occur, but usually stops rapidly. If haemorrhage persists and obstructs the surgical view, one or two drops of neutral adrenaline 1/1000 or 1/10 000 will usually stop the bleeding.

POSTOPERATIVE CARE

Patients are discharged very soon after surgery, but the eye should be kept padded until the following day. From that time on, guttae chloramphenicol and guttae prednisolone 0.3% or 0.5% are instilled three times a day for 2 weeks. After this time no further medication should be required. Patients should be asked to attend for follow-up at 2 weeks, 6 weeks and 12 weeks, and all patients should have been warned preoperatively that the final refractive results of the surgery will not be known until 3 months after the operation, at which time consideration can be given to the desirability or necessity of surgery for the other eye.

POSTOPERATIVE COMPLICATIONS

Undercorrection

Undercorrection is the commonest of the undesired refractive results following radial keratotomy. For patients who have already had eight incisions, the best advice seems to be to encourage the patient to accept the situation, rather than to double the amount of surgical pathology for what will always be a meagre return. The second eight incisions will only increase the correction by a small proportion of what has already been achieved. For patients who have had four incisions only, a further four may usefully be added, though this is best left until at least 6 months after the first procedure. Certainly, a minimum period of 3 months must always elapse between two procedures.

Overcorrection

Overcorrection is a less common, but always unwelcome complication. Great care must be taken with patients in the older age group, to do less surgery for their degree of myopia than would be required for younger subjects.

Loss of binocular vision

Radial keratotomy is occasionally undertaken for the management of myopic anisometropia, even where the more myopic eye may be relatively amblyopic. The object of the operation is to reduce the strength of the correction needed for the more myopic eye in an effort to equalize the two eyes. Unfortunately, for patients who already have good binocular vision despite their anisometropia, alteration of the refraction can result in loss of binocular vision. This can be important in patients whose binocular single vision is an important requirement for their work.

Diurnal variation of refraction

Most patients find that their myopia is more corrected, or even overcorrected, on rising in the morning, and that the degree of correction or overcorrection is significantly reduced in the evening. Most patients are able to tolerate this nuisance without difficulty, and the problem usually subsides after several weeks or months. Occasionally, however, the symptom can be persistent. The symptom is attributed to the weakened structure of the cornea, which probably alters its curvature during the day in line with altered stromal hydration.

Nocturnal glare or 'starburst' effect

Patients may find that in poor light, e.g. at night, when the pupil is dilated, point sources of illumination may take on streak distortions, or may produce an effect whereby the patient can actually perceive the corneal incisions within the pupillary area. These symptoms are seldom so severe as to be disabling, but this can occasionally be the case. Strangely, some patients are never aware of this problem, while others are bothered by it for a long period.

Infection

Patients whose surgery is carried out under sterile conditions and followed by appropriate postoperative care are unlikely to develop infections as a direct result of the surgery in the early postoperative period. All patients, however, who have undergone radial keratotomy are at long-term risk of deep-seated keratitis, due to infective organisms lodging at the base of the corneal incisions. All patients must be warned of this complication so that they will seek early treatment in the event of symptoms developing. These risks of infection are, of course, greatly increased when patients have associated contributory factors, such as diabetes mellitus, chronic lid margin disease or the wearing of contact lenses after radial keratotomy. Patients developing acute keratitis in an eye which has previously undergone radial keratotomy should be admitted to hospital for investigation and intensive medical management. Failure to manage this complication has resulted in permanent loss of vision.

Long-term instability of refractive result

As years have now passed since the introduction of radial keratotomy, it has become recognized that a proportion of patients undergo a degree of reinforcement of the original effect of the surgery; thus patients left emmetropic may gradually become hypermetropic, and patients left undercorrected may gradually suffer or enjoy a slow reduction of the residual myopia towards emmetropia. The full extent to which this process may extend, or its duration, is not yet fully identified.

Mini-RK

In recent years, some refractive surgeons have modified their radial keratotomy technique to perform a mini-RK. These incisions are much shorter than those described above, each incision being no more than 2–3.5 mm long and towards the corneal periphery (Fig 21.5). Again, such incisions have to be placed as deep as possible if they are to achieve the desired correction. It has been found that mini incisions of this sort can correct low degrees of myopia just as efficiently as the longer incisions. The advantage is that the complication rate is reduced. Surgeons report a reduced incidence of preoperative perforation and reduced problems with postoperative diurnal variation. The basic problems, however, of a weakened cornea with incisions which never really heal to restore the original corneal integrity and the long-term

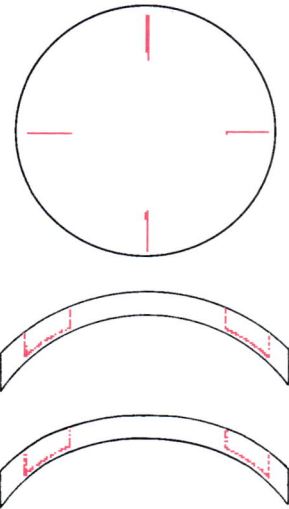

Fig. 21.5.

risks of infection do remain even with this reduced level of corneal trauma. The authors of this chapter have limited experience with this technique, but where it has been used for the correction of very low levels of myopia, it has been found to be highly effective.

22

Epikeratoplasty

Although epikeratoplasty has been practised for several years it should still be regarded as an experimental technique. As yet it has not reached a degree of refinement which would permit an accurately predictable outcome.

INDICATIONS

There are two major indications: firstly, the correction of high spherical refractive errors in the absence of any other suitable means, e.g. contact lens or secondary lens implant; and secondly, the correction of some cases of keratoconus. In keratoconus, a plano lens is used to flatten the cone and eliminate the irregular astigmatism. For epikeratoplasty to be feasible, there must be no scarring or opacity in the visual axis. In any situation where rapid correction of vision is necessary, e.g. in early infancy to prevent amblyopia, epikeratoplasty is not ideal since it may take some months for the applied tissue lens to clear.

SURGICAL TECHNIQUE

Corneal tissue lenses may be obtained commercially or may be manufactured on a cryolathe from a donor eye; the techniques involved are beyond the scope of this manual. Preoperative pilocarpine drops may help to centre the trephine.

1. Superior and inferior rectus sutures are used to fix the eye so that it is looking directly forwards.

2. The epithelium must be removed from the central cornea for a diameter of 8–9 mm. This is best done with a scalpel blade (Bard Parker D15) wiping with gentle sweeps across the corneal surface (Fig. 22.1). When all the central epithelium appears to have been removed, the surface should be wiped with a cellulose sponge moistened with alcohol to ensure that there will be no viable cells in the interface between host and 'epi' button. Failure to do this

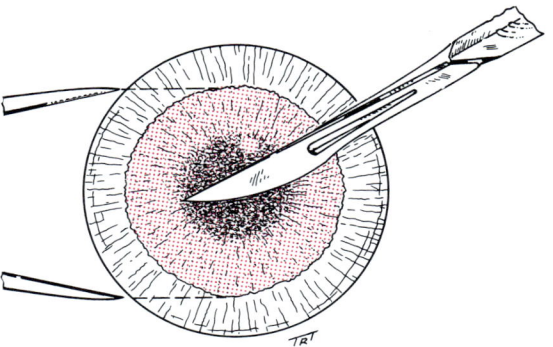

Fig. 22.1.

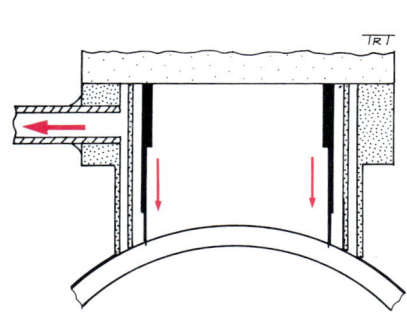

Fig. 22.2.

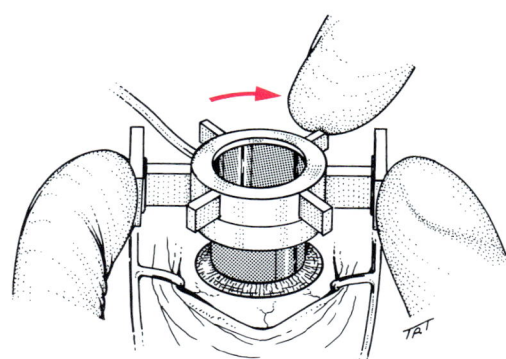

Fig. 22.3.

adequately can lead to interface opacity and may necessitate the removal of the 'epi'.

The cornea should be washed with saline to remove any residual debris.

3. The cornea must now be carefully marked so that the lens will be centred accurately on the visual axis. The trephine can be lightly pressed against the surface of the cornea until the correct position is found. A Hessburg–Baron suction trephine (Figs 22.2 and 22.3) should be used, since this can deliver a very precise cut. It also has crosswires which help in centring.

4. Suction is applied and the trephine turned for three quarter turns (Fig. 22.3). This cuts to a depth of 0.075 mm.

5. Next, stroma must be undermined peripherally at this depth to make a pocket to hold the wing of the lens. A 23 gauge needle bent back at the bevel to $120°$ can be inserted into the depth of the trephine cut, and gradually swept round through $360°$ (Fig. 22.4).

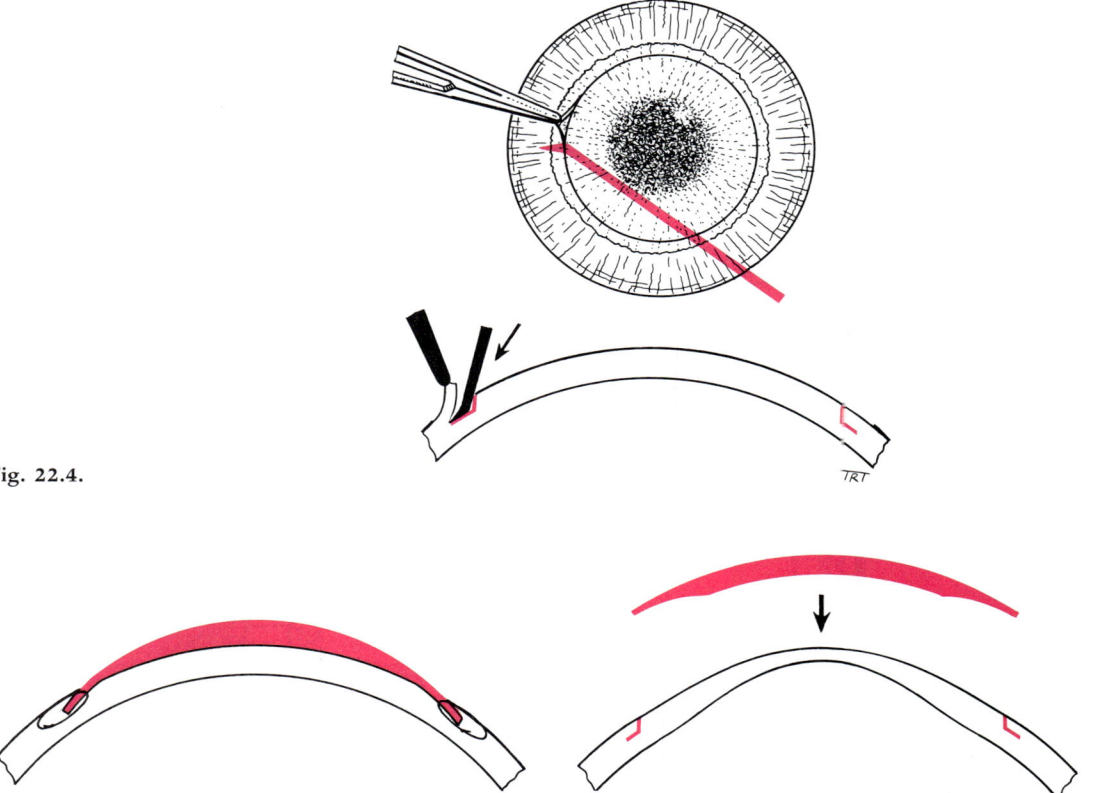

Fig. 22.4.

Fig. 22.5.

Fig. 22.6.

This should provide an adequate pocket for the wing but, if necessary, it can be deepened later.

6. If a dessicated lens is being used, it should be rehydrated.

7. Using 10/0 nylon (unless the indication is for keratoconus), the lens is sutured in place using 8 or 12 interrupted sutures. The suture is passed fully through the edge of the optic of the lens, and then into the pocket in the stroma out on to the corneal surface and tied (Fig. 22.5).

8. After all the sutures are tied, the wing can be tucked into the pocket with an iris repositor. At this stage it is wise to check that there is not undue tension on any of the sutures producing astigmatism. A Maloney keratometer is adequate for this. Any overtight sutures should be replaced. Finally, the knots are buried.

9. In the case of keratoconus (Fig. 22.6) the technique is substantially the same, but 9/0 nylon is used since the sutures must be tight so that the lens compresses the cornea. Once the first suture is

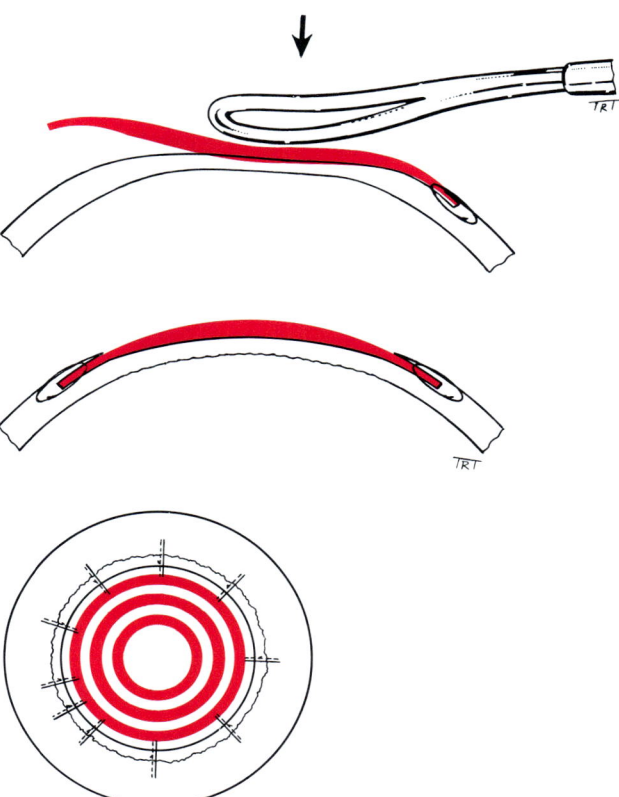

Fig. 22.7.

Fig. 22.8.

Fig. 22.9.

inserted, the sutures are inserted in opposite quadrants and the assistant compresses the cornea (with a spatula or vectis) while the surgeon tightens the suture (Figs 22.7 and 22.8). In this situation astigmatism is easily produced, and care must be taken that the end result is as nearly spherical as possible before the surgery ends. Again, meticulous care with the use of keratometry is essential if undue astigmatism is to be avoided. This may involve changing several sutures or inserting additional ones (Fig. 22.9).

10. A subconjunctival injection of antibiotic is given at the end of the procedure, and afterwards topical steroid and antibiotics are given for a few weeks. The eye need only be padded until the following morning.

POSTOPERATIVE CARE

Care may need to be taken with removal of the sutures in the case of keratoconus, since excess astigmatism may be induced (Fig. 22.10). In all

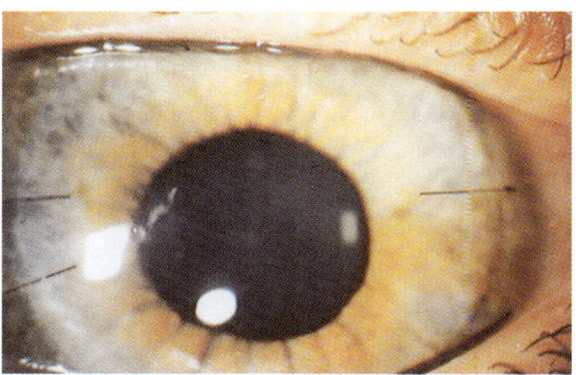

Fig. 22.10.

cases sutures should be left *in situ* for as long as possible, consistent with optical requirements.

Removal of the lens is easy (it peels off) and may be required for interface opacity, e.g. due to residual epithelial cells, for infection or for grossly inaccurate refractive correction.

COMPLICATIONS

A grossly inaccurate correction may be produced, in which case the lens may have to be replaced.

The epithelium may fail to heal adequately. Using fresh, cryolathed tissue, re-epithelialization is not a problem. The commercially prepared material does occasionally lead to slow epithelial healing, and a bandage contact lens or tarsorraphy may be indicated. Filamentary keratitis (wet type) may also be encountered. The filaments may be gently debrided and acetyl cysteine drops used. A bandage contact lens may also be needed for a few weeks until the epithelium stabilizes.

Like any other form of keratoplasty, loosening of the sutures may be found. Any loose sutures should be removed.

Interface opacities occasionally develop. These are usually due to replication of epithelial cells left behind on Bowman's membrane. The opacification may be sufficient to reduce vision greatly, and is usually enough to warrant removal of the 'epi'.

Infection in the lens has been reported from time to time and, again, is usually an indication to remove the lens.

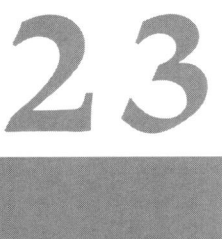

Excimer laser photorefractive keratectomy (PRK) (corneal reprofiling)

At the time of the preparation of the original first edition of this book, excimer laser surgery was still in its earliest experimental stages. Since that time, the procedure has been performed on many thousands of patients, but even at this time, the procedure is being continually refined in order to improve the success rate, and to eliminate the established disadvantages. A chapter on this subject is included in this book for the purposes of completion, but the authors would wish to stress that the information contained in this chapter should not be deemed to replace a proper training instruction for surgeons wishing to use this technique upon patients. The technique described, therefore, will be a rough outline only to include the current principles involved.

INDICATIONS

Theoretically, excimer laser reprofiling is applicable to a wide range of refractive errors, including hypermetropia, myopia and astigmatism. By far the greatest experience is with the treatment of myopia and astigmatism. Currently, PRK is regarded as a satisfactory technique for patients with low myopia perhaps up to 6 or 8 dioptres. It has been found that although the technique can be used for people with higher degrees of myopia, the success rate falls away progressively as the pre-operative myopic error increases, and it is probable that for these higher degrees of myopia, alternative techniques will prove to be more reliable. Experience with PRK for the treatment of astigmatism usually associated with myopia has shown that for the low degrees of astigmatism, satisfactory results can be achieved, though the results are very variable. Certainly, increasing astigmatic powers are associated with falling success rates.

The management of hypermetropia by PRK is still in its infancy, but the principles will be examined. At the time of writing, successful results have been obtained for up to 4 dioptres of hypermetropia.

It is the authors' belief that all patients enquiring about laser refractive procedures should be advised that these refractive techniques are best regarded as experimental and unpredictable. The limits of the procedures are not yet clearly established, nor has the range of possible complications been fully identified. Long-term effects and the stability of the refractive results of these procedures remain to be determined.

INSTRUMENTS

A number of excimer lasers suitable for corneal reprofiling are currently on the market. Results for various models are variable, and prospective purchasers are well advised to consider all the relevant literature. These lasers deliver a laser beam of 193 nm with a pulse frequency of 6 to 10 Hz. The delivery system of each machine permits individual laser cuts to be of a depth no greater than 0.2 μ. This refinement provides a very high degree of control for the surgeon. The underlying physical principles connected with the excimer laser are beyond the scope of this text.

PATIENT PREPARATION

The most important part of the preoperative preparation for any patient undergoing laser refractive surgery is thorough counselling. In the light of the presenting refractive error, the surgeon should be able to provide the patient with a reasonable assessment of the likely postoperative outcome. Care should be taken to make patients well aware of the fact that there are complications following these procedures, some of which are prejudicial to good vision. These procedures are still the subject of investigation and it is the authors' opinion that patients should be aware of this. Surgeons should take care to ensure that no intending patient is under the impression that there can be any guarantee of a successful or problem-free outcome. Patients should certainly be warned that laser treatment is often followed by severe pain which may last for several days in the worst cases. They also need to be aware that the intended refractive outcome is not obtained immediately, and may not be established for some months after the laser procedure.

PREOPERATIVE MEDICATION

It is no longer considered essential for laser patients to have constricted pupils before the procedure.

SURGICAL TECHNIQUE

Anaesthesia

A few minutes before the delivery of the laser, drops of topical anaesthesia are administered to the eye to be treated. Amethocaine or benoxinate are usually employed. Retrobulbar or peribulbar injections are not required. The patient needs to retain full control of eye movement. Similarly, a facial block is not required.

Instructions to the patient

Laser reprofiling requires a high degree of patient cooperation. The patient focuses on a target light within the laser beam and, for accuracy of beam placement, the patient needs to be able to maintain fixation throughout the period of treatment. Minor fluctuations attributable to microsaccades do not appear to prejudice a satisfactory outcome. The patient needs to understand the importance of maintaining fixation.

A light wire speculum is inserted on the side to be treated and the other eye is either padded or covered with an occlusive shield to assist the patient in fixating the eye undergoing treatment.

Epithelial removal

The patient is first accurately aligned under the laser beam. During treatment, the laser is applied to Bowman's membrane and the under-lying stroma. It is, therefore, necessary for the overlying epithelium to be removed before the refractive treatment. A number of techniques can be used for this which include manual debridement (Fig. 23.1), total laser removal or a combination of the two referred to as 'laser scrape'. With this technique which the authors prefer, the anterior 40 µm are removed with the laser and the remaining epithelium on the surface of Bowman's membrane can be lightly brushed away with a cellulose swab (Fig. 23.2). The advantages of this technique are:

1. Bowman's membrane remains untouched.

2. No more epithelium than is absolutely necessary is disturbed.

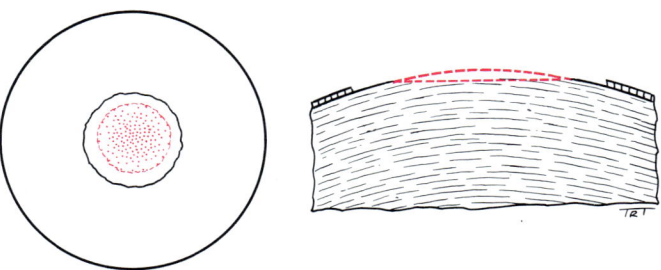

Fig. 23.1.

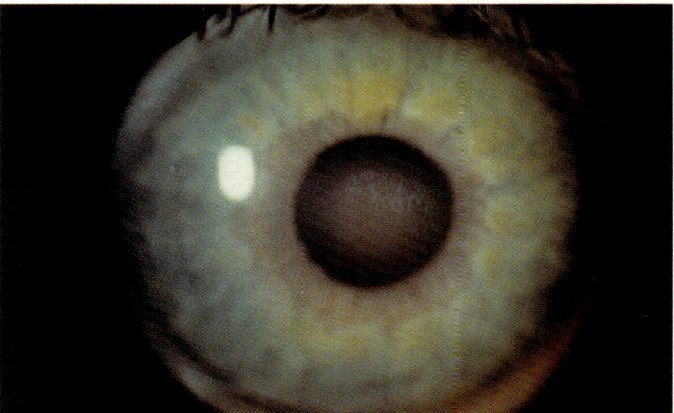

Fig. 23.2.

3. The outline of the epithelium removed will correspond to the treating laser beam and accuracy of centration can therefore be checked before the final treatment commences.

Laser treatment

Refractive lasers are controlled by computers and the patient's data are carefully and accurately entered into the program. As soon as the computer indicates that the laser has been appropriately armed, the area for corneal reprofiling is carefully dried. With the patient maintaining steady fixation under microscopic control from the laser operator, the beam is applied to produce the necessary correction. The period of treatment will vary depending upon the degree of correction to be achieved and most treatments take 10–40 seconds.

Dressing

Following treatment, the eye is dressed using antibiotics and non-steroidal anti-inflammatory agents associated with a firm pad. In view of the fact that the patient is likely to experience pain during the first postoperative day, particularly after the local anaesthesia has worn off, suitable analgesia needs to be provided. Some units routinely fit the patient with a soft bandage contact lens which is left in place until the epithelium has recovered the treatment area. The use of these contact lenses, however, is controversial. The eyes are more comfortable, but the risks of infection are increased.

POSTOPERATIVE CARE

During experimental clinical trials, patients are seen at regular intervals and their progress carefully documented. The epithelium usually heals after 2 or 3 days and after this time the eye should no longer be painful or uncomfortable. There is sometimes an alteration of refraction to hypermetropia, though this is less marked with some of the more modern lasers. This change, however, is brief only and has usually totally disappeared within 2–4 weeks. The refraction gradually stabilizes within the first 3 months of postoperative treatment, but in some cases instability persists for longer. After 6 weeks or so, it is not uncommon to note some degree of anterior stromal haze in the treated area. This complication was originally described as 'always transient', but, in fact, proved in some cases to be nothing of the sort. In some patients, the corneal haze alters to become corneal scarring, persisting for some years after treatment. Newer laser systems and refinements in understanding and software have reduced this complication. The use of steroid medication topically, originally deemed to be essential, has now been shown to have no useful long-term benefit for laser refractive patients, and the use has fallen into disrepute because of the distorted refractive results which the use of steroid can produce, and because of the significant incidence of steroid-induced glaucoma.

COMPLICATIONS

The list of complications reported following PRK is now extensive. At the time of writing this chapter for the first edition, it was stated that no sight-threatening complications had been reported. This is no longer true. Sight-threatening problems may occur, albeit rarely, and they include:

1. surface and stromal keratopathy in patients with connective tissue disease;
2. laser induced/activated herpetic keratitis; and
3. bacterial keratitis, usually associated with the postoperative use of bandage contact lenses.

Persisting corneal haze (Fig. 23.3) is certainly reported, and is associated with reduced visual acuity and reduced contrast sensitivity. In cases where this is associated with a dramatic alteration of refractive power, patients may lose binocular function. More common complications would include undercorrection and overcorrection, together with inconvenient alteration of astigmatic power. The worst of these is the induction of an irregular component which will prevent a patient achieving good uncorrected or spectacle corrected vision and, therefore, necessitating either contact lens wear or re-treatment. The incidence of most complications, however, is being progressively reduced by

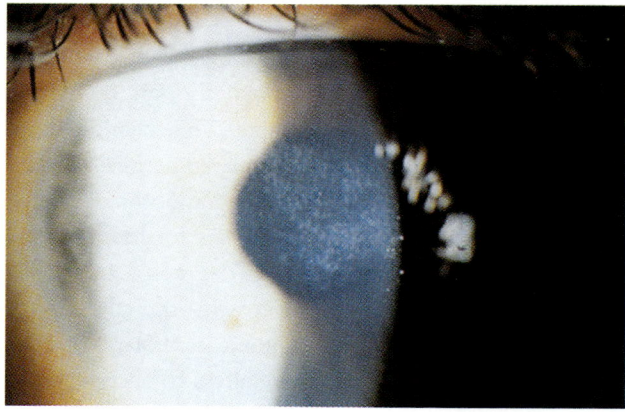

Fig. 23.3.

improvement in laser systems and their related software. Reduced contrast sensitivity, however, causing poor quality of vision in poor light, persists indefinitely for some, despite the absence of demonstrable corneal opacity.

One further point about intraocular pressure and the dangers of glaucoma is worth making. All early patients following PRK were treated with topical steroid, and this use of steroid is still commonly practised. At least 10% of patients taking regular topical steroid are at risk of developing steroid glaucoma. A measurement of intraocular pressure by applanation tonometry, however, is rendered inaccurate by the PRK technique and particularly for patients where higher degrees of correction have been attempted. The loss of stroma and Descemet's membrane together makes it possible to record relatively low levels of intraocular pressure in patients where the pressure is actually considerably higher. Practitioners need to be aware of this potential hazard.

PRK for hypermetropia

This technique is in its very earliest experimental stages, but the principle of the technique is illustrated in Figure 23.4. By removing an annulus of peripheral corneal tissue, the central curvature can be increased, thereby correcting hypermetropia.

RESULTS

Good early results for low hypermetropes of between 1 and 4 dioptres have been reported. No reliable data for long-term results of this form of treatment are currently available. It is, however, known that refractive techniques for hypermetropia have been plagued by early

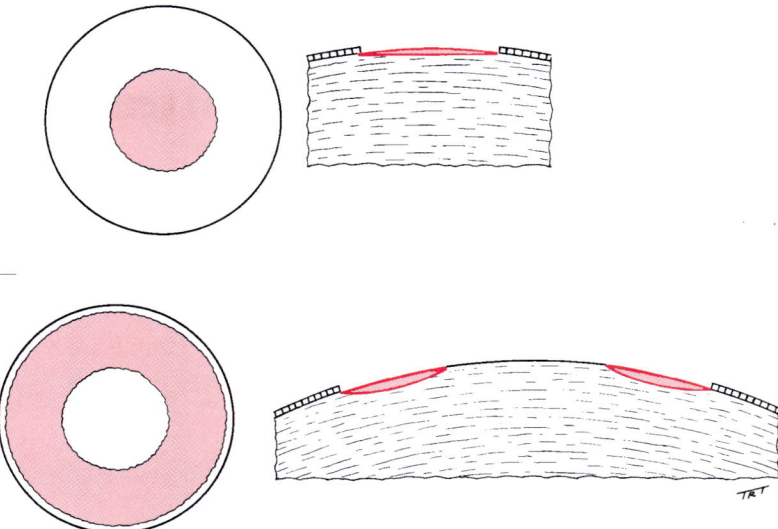

Fig. 23.4.

satisfactory results which then are followed by regression. It remains to be seen whether PRK patients will fare better in this respect.

24 Lamellar refractive surgical techniques

HISTORICAL BACKGROUND

In the late 1940s and the years that followed, a Spanish surgeon, Jose Barraquer, working in Colombia, devised two lamellar surgical procedures which could be used for the correction of myopia and hypermetropia. For myopia (Fig. 24.1) the technique was called keratomileusis. This operation comprised the removal of a layer of the central cornea of approximately 8 mm in diameter and of perhaps half corneal thickness. This was achieved with a microkeratome. The microkeratome consisted of an oscillating blade mounted in a cutting head which crossed the cornea which, in turn, was secured by a suction ring. The oscillating blade passed across the top of the suction ring along guiderails. The corneal disc so obtained was then frozen and mounted on a cryolathe. Following careful calculation, a positive stromal lens was lathed away from the undersurface of the disc which was then thawed and returned to the surface of the cornea.

The operation of keratophakia for the correction of hypermetropia (Fig. 24.2) involved the removal of a similar disc of corneal tissue and in

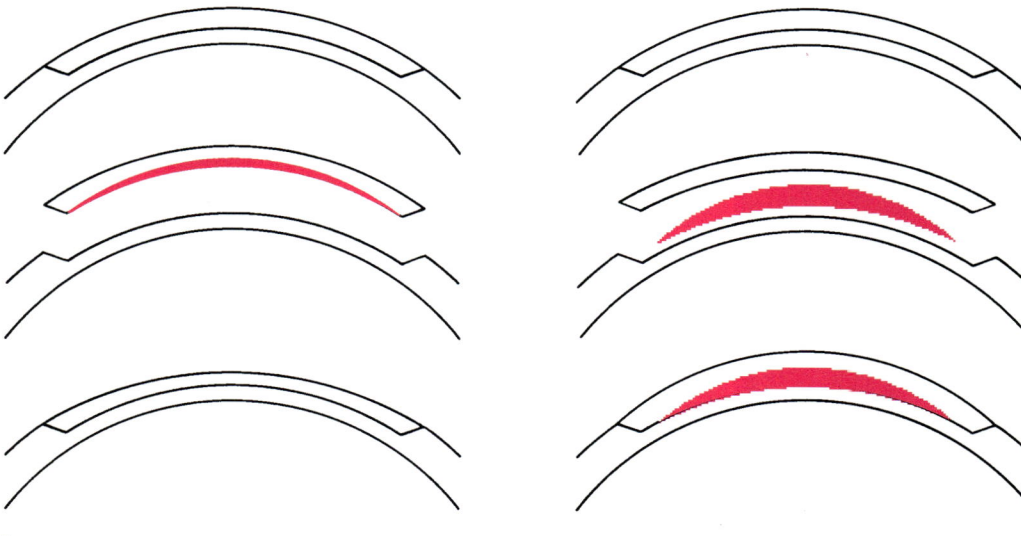

Fig. 24.1.   Fig. 24.2.

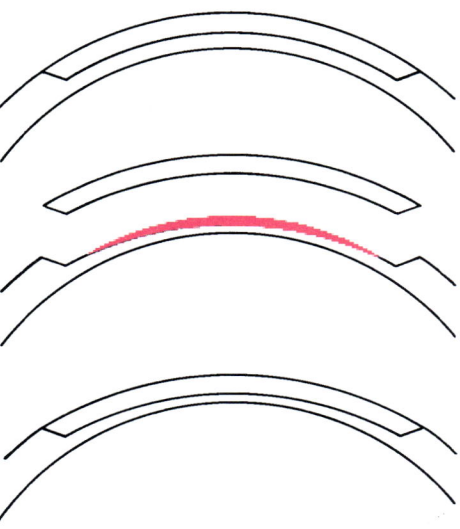

Fig. 24.3.

this case a positive lens of donor stromal material was obtained from a donor cornea and this positive disc was then placed within the patient's stroma sandwiched between the two layers of cornea achieved by the microkeratome.

While excellent results for keratomileusis and keratophakia were reported by Barraquer, the techniques were always extremely complicated and beyond the scope of most ophthalmic practitioners. Epikeratophakia as discussed in Chapter 22 is one of the offshoots of the procedures devised by Barraquer. Because of the technical difficulties associated with the treatment of the higher refractive errors with PRK, several lamellar techniques have been devised as alternatives:

1. Automated lamellar keratoplasty (ALK)

The only difference between this surgical procedure and keratomileusis as devised by Barraquer is that instead of using a cryolathe to remove a predetermined lens of stromal tissue from the superficial lamella, ALK uses a modified microkeratome to remove a similar lens of stromal tissue from the cut stromal surface as illustrated in Figure 24.3. The microkeratome for this technique is even more complicated than that devised by Barraquer. Although enthusiastic practitioners reported encouraging results, where laser surgical alternatives have been permitted and available, ALK has failed to generate a large following.

For satisfactory patients, however, the advantages of the technique were the absence of significant scarring and relatively rapid visual rehabilitation compared with PRK. Complications included corneal perforation, overcorrection, undercorrection, opacities at the interface and infection.

2. Laser keratomileusis

For a brief period, Buratto in Italy and others used this technique for the management of higher levels of myopia. A microkeratome was used to obtain a disc of stromal tissue approximately 8 mm in diameter and of one-half to two-thirds stromal depth. The posterior surface of the lamellar disc was then taken to the laser and centred under the treatment beam. An appropriate correcting ablation was then applied to the posterior surface of the disc which was then re-sutured to the cornea. The advantage of this technique over PRK was the ability to treat higher degrees of refractive error, the absence of anterior stromal haze and a rapid visual rehabilitation. The problems, however, were the same as those for the original procedure, namely refractive problems related to decentration, particularly for higher corrections and the development of opacities at the interface in the mid stroma.

3. Laser assisted in situ keratomileusis (LASIK)

This is the most recent development of lamellar refractive techniques and has been devised by Pallikaris. The difference between this technique and laser keratomileusis as mentioned above is, firstly, that the stromal flap is not removed completely, but is hinged either nasally or superiorly, and, secondly, that the laser ablation is applied to the exposed stromal surface beneath the flap (Fig. 24.4). The advantages of this technique are the increased speed and convenience of the procedure

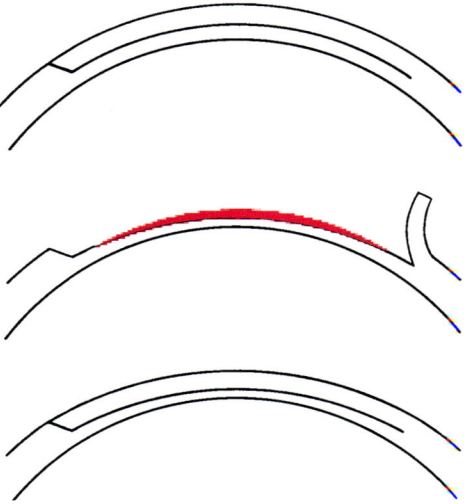

Fig. 24.4.

which can now be conducted with the patient lying under the laser beam. The hinged flap is immediately returned to position after the application of the laser and requires no suturing. In practised hands, this technique is swift and sure though the learning curve is associated with a number of well-documented complications which include loss of the flap, perforation of the anterior chamber, over-correction, under-correction, decentration and the same problems with opacities at the interface and the risks of infection. The advantages, however, are the speed of the procedure, the absence of pain for the patient, the speed of visual rehabilitation and the increased range of initial refractive errors which can be safely tackled.

Theoretically, lamellar refractive surgery is an attractive idea and the advantages of a wider range of corrective possibilities and rapid visual rehabilitation are significant. The technical difficulties associated with the techniques, however, will restrict their widespread adoption. It is, as yet, too soon to be sure of the quality of the refractive outcome. Patient numbers are not large.

Alternatively, PRK is a simpler technique with a rising success rate, even for higher refractive errors. The eventual place of the relationship between the separate approaches is not yet finalized.

Further reading

Section A

Rabinowitz, Y. S., Wilson, S. E. and Klyce, S. D. (1993). *Color Atlas of Corneal Topography*. Igaku-Shoin, New York.

Wilson, S. E., Klyce, S. D. and Husseini, Z. M. (1993). Standardized color-coded maps for corneal topography. *Opthalmology*, **100**, 1723–7.

Section B

Chell, P. B., Hope Ross, M. W., Shah, P. and McDonnell, P. J. (1996). Long-term follow-up of a single continuous adjustable suture penetrating keratoplasty. *Eye*, **10**, 133–7.

Claoue, C., Flicker, L., Kirkness, C. and Steele, A. (1993). Refractive results after corneal triple procedures (PK + ECCE + IOL). *Eye*, **7**, 466–51.

Filatov, V., Alexandrakis, G., Talamo, J. H. and Steinert, R. F. (1996). Comparison of suture-in and suture-out post-keratoplasty astigmatism with single running suture or combined running and interrupted sutures. *Am. J. Ophthalmol.*, **122**, 696–700.

Kirkness, C. M., Ling, Y. and Rice, N. S. C. (1988). The use of silicone drainage tubing in the management of post-keratoplasty glaucoma. *Eye*, **2**, 583–90.

Kirkness, C. M., Flicker, L. A., Steele, A. D. McG. and Rice, N. S. C. (1991). The role of penetrating keratoplasty in the management of microbial keratitis. *Eye*, **5**, 425–31.

Kirkness, C. M., Steele, A. D. McG., Ficker, L. A. and Rice, N. S. C. (1992). The management of coexistent glaucoma by combined penetrating keratoplasty and trabeculectomy or trabeculectomy and subsequent surgery. *Br. J. Ophthalmol.*, **76**, 156–68.

Mader, T. H., Yuan, R., Lynn, M. J., Stulting, R. D., Wilson, L. A. and Waring, G. O. 3rd (1993). Changes in keratometric astigmatism after suture removal more than one year after penetrating keratoplasty. *Ophthalmology*, **100**, 119–26.

Serdarevic, O. N., Renard, G. J. and Pouliquen, Y. (1994). Randomized clinical trial comparing astigmatism and visual rehabilitation after penetrating keratoplasty with and without intraoperative suture adjustment. *Ophthalmology*, **101**, 990–9.

Section C

Kirkness, C. M., Adams, G. G. W., Dilly, N. P. and Lee, J. P. (1988). Botulinum toxin A induced protective ptosis in the management of corneal disease. *Ophthalmology*, **95**, 473–80.

Kirkness, C. M., Ficker, L. A., Steele, A. D. McG. and Rice, N. S. C. (1991). Graft-refractive surgery after penetrating keratoplasty for keratoconus. *Ophthalmology*. **98**, 1786–92.

Leahey, A. B., Gottsch, J. D. and Stark, W. J. (1993). Clinical experience with N-butyl cyanoacrylate (Nexacryl) tissue adhesive. *Ophthalmology*, **100**, 173–80.

Riordan, E. P., Kielhorn, I., Ficker, L. A., Steele, A. D. and Kirkness, C. M. (1993). Conjunctival autografting in the surgical management of pterygium. *Eye*, **7**, 634–8.

Wagoner, M. D., Kenyon, K. R. and Shore, J. W. (1995). Ocular surface transplantation. In: *Recent Advances in Ophthalmology* (Jay, B., Kirkness, C. M., eds). Churchill Livingston, London.

Section D

Ficker, L. A., Bates, A. K., Steele, A. D. *et al.*, (1993). Excimer laser photorefractive keratectomy for myopia; 12 month follow-up. *Eye*, **7**, 617–24.

Kirkness, C. M., Ficker, L. A., Steele, A. D. McG. and Rice, N. S. C. (1991). Graft-refractive surgery after penetrating keratoplasty for keratoconus. *Ophthalmology*. **98**, 1786–92.

Waring, G. O. 3rd, Lynn, M. J. and McDonnell, P. J. (1994). Results of the prospective evaluation of radial keratomy (PERK) study 10 years after surgery. *Arch. Ophthalmol.*, **112**, 1298–308.

Index